A MID-LIFE LESS ORDINARY

A MID-LIFE LESS ORDINARY

From Ultramarathon Insanity
to Rowing the Atlantic at Fifty

PETER WRIGHT
with Steve Wright

First published by Pitch Publishing, 2025

1

Pitch Publishing
9 Donnington Park,
85 Birdham Road,
Chichester, West Sussex,
PO20 7AJ

www.pitchpublishing.co.uk
info@pitchpublishing.co.uk

A CIP catalogue record is available for this book
from the British Library.

ISBN 978 1 80150 965 7

Typesetting and origination by Pitch Publishing

Printed and bound in the UK on FSC® certified paper in line
with our continuing commitment to ethical business practices,
sustainability and the environment.

Printed and bound by CPI Group (UK) Ltd, Croydon, CR0 4YY

Contents

To my wonderful wife, Rach, and my two children, Josh and Leila. Without your constant support, there would be little content for this book.

Also, to my dad for loaning us the cash to get the rowing dream started and for meeting me in Antigua. Finding out mid-row that you would be there was just the lift I needed. I will cherish that time spent together.

Editor's note

WE ALL have a story to tell. And as strange as it may sound, considering that Pete's my brother, it was really only after sitting down with him on numerous occasions while making plans for this book that I truly appreciated just *how much* of a story he has to tell.

There's a fairly big age gap between us – 15 years – so during my early years, he seemed more like the cool uncle than an older brother. We've always had a strong dynamic, and as I got older, the more brotherly relationship came to the fore, fermented during boozy weekends in Jersey and watching AFC Bournemouth's improbable rise up the leagues.

When Pete ran in the London Marathon for the first time, that seemed like a big thing. Later on, the Marathon des Sables seemed almost unfathomable in its difficulty. By the time the Jungle Marathon came around, his mates and I were predicting what tropical-themed fatality would await him in the Amazon.

It wasn't that I wasn't impressed by his endeavours; it was impossible not to be in awe of him. One year, Pete bought me entry to the Bournemouth Marathon as a birthday present (I'd have probably preferred money, to be honest), and ran alongside me (it's fair to say that he slowed down for me!). Using this as my benchmark – and how utterly, utterly shattered I was after crawling across the finish line, Pete having kept me company the entire way – what he was doing seemed superhuman. But there were so many challenges that it was a challenge in itself to keep track of them, let alone appreciate all the finer details.

Seeing Pete and Steve set off from La Gomera to traverse the Atlantic, however, it was impossible not to look at the finer details. This tiny boat would be their home for the better part of two months. They wouldn't sleep for any longer than two hours at a time. Moreover, they'd essentially be alone, a long way from the help of even the support boat. 'Humbled' couldn't have been more inadequate a feeling.

Before and during Pete's discovery of his enduring passion for pushing himself to the limit, I was embarking on my own career in publishing. I've been fortunate enough to work with some very talented people across several great titles. So when Pete asked me for my assistance in putting his story together, it was great to know that I could help out in some small way.

While we already had a good relationship, the process of writing this book has undoubtedly helped me to understand Pete better, both in terms of his achievements, and the mindset that has paved the way towards them.

Beyond that, his story can serve as a positive case study for anyone who wants more out of life. Pete's approach has always been one of throwing himself into things, aided by careful preparation, with the odd setback only providing a lesson for future endeavours and fuel for bouncing back. These approaches are far from rocket science, but the results could genuinely be life-altering.

Taken on its own basis, however, this is purely an account of one man who kept pushing to see how far he can go, and so far hasn't stopped! I hope you enjoy reading this as much as we did putting it together.

Steve Wright

Foreword

OVER THE last 30 years, I've run over 1,100 marathons, set nine Guinness World Records for endurance running on treadmills, and completed the Marathon des Sables 17 times. I feel very fortunate to have been able to have such an extended and rewarding athletic career that, luckily for me, has become my vocation. I now coach people the world over to achieve their personal bests and achieve their dreams.

It wasn't always like that – in my earlier existence, I was addicted to alcohol and nicotine, and had little life direction or hope of a brighter future. Back in 1994, you didn't reach out for help; you just got on with things and didn't complain. I'd now be identified as severely depressed, and it would be seen as being a strong thing to seek professional support, rather than a sign of embarrassing weakness. My life back then was very different.

But then came a lifestyle shift, and on 5 January 1994, for some unaccountable reason, I felt that I needed to go for a run. After my first outing of 100 lung-busting strides, I'd found my salvation – the exoskeleton that would support my daily life forever. Suddenly, I had a fresh direction and a new purpose, and in a few short months my life became super-positive. I stopped drinking and smoking, and concentrated on becoming healthier.

As my running career progressed, and the distances I could run grew longer, the challenges grew as well. The Marathon des Sables beckoned, and in 1999 I ran the race for the first time. It has become part of my DNA, and the MDS is part of my everyday world.

Over the years, I've coached thousands of people to run the MDS. I first met Pete in October 2012, six months prior to the 28th edition of the race in April 2013. I was immediately struck by his enthusiasm and dedication to the training, especially as he had to travel over from Jersey to Cardiff to engage with me on a one-to-one session to begin his MDS immersion process. His approach was perfect, as the best way to get ready for any challenge is to find a person that has already paid the price both physically and mentally for what you want to achieve, and Pete became a great MDS apprentice.

Following a day of gym tests and a marathon along the Welsh Coast Path together, I knew Pete had exactly what it would take to finish the MDS and go on to undertake the many future life challenges he had planned. Determination is his key driver, and failure isn't an option. The whole process of learning new aptitudes has provided the momentum to succeed and take on even greater feats.

Overcoming the problems experienced in both training and the event itself really helps when life throws a curveball. This happened to me in 2016 when I was paralysed with Guillain-Barré Syndrome, a rare neurological condition that challenged my very existence. Having to learn to walk again took an immense amount of determination, and, luckily for me, there are no long-lasting effects of my being so ill.

I identified that same determination when I met Pete. The MDS proved to be a great introduction to the world of extreme feats, and I've followed his progress with great interest when he completed his Smart-car marathon, and then when he went on to row the Atlantic. It's amazing what he's achieved following the changes he made in 2012.

We all have the ability to change; to change every aspect of our lives. However, actually making those changes and having the courage to make those changes requires three things: bravery, daring and a dash of audacity – all of which I see in Peter Wright.

Like everyone else that knows Pete, I'm waiting with bated breath to see what his next challenge will be. I wish him every success in the future.

Rory Coleman

Prologue

EVERYONE'S GOT a preferred way to enjoy the festive period. Generally, it will involve a lot of spending time with loved ones, plenty of cheer, watching TV and invariably relaxing and doing things that aren't particularly taxing.

Now, I knew that this was not how this particular Christmas was going to be, but I really wasn't expecting to be in the predicament I'm currently in.

Instead, I'm confined to a cabin only just long enough to accommodate my 6ft body length. The treasured gifts of small cheeses and a mini-bottle of wine that I'd received from my wife, Rachel, have been washed away overboard. I try to lie still and get some sleep – easier said than done when the cabin rocks from side to side, not always with reliable regularity, sea sickness kept at bay only by some handy tablets.

As I roll over in an attempt to get comfortable, a renegade wave catches the boat and sends me face-first into the ship's radio. My skin uncomfortably peels off the plastic interior of the cabin that has been my home for the last couple of weeks – a cabin that has come to resemble a sweat box.

Distractions are few and far between – earlier on in the voyage, we had speakers to blare out rousing music from the iPod, an iPad to watch downloaded movies, and a Kindle for a bit of light reading. As it turns out, such devices don't last very long in environments with a lot of moisture. In this cabin, there's plenty of that to go around.

Amid all this, while I dream wistfully of pigs in blankets and Boxing Day football, I have one distraction: my crewmate, Steve, who's lying across from – or, more accurately, right next to – me, playing the harmonica while completely naked.

Exiting the cabin to go out on deck is out of the question – the force of the winds battering us makes any kind of progress impossible. For situations like this, there's a drogue (a type of sea anchor) that can be deployed, which gives us a bit of stability and stops the boat from being blown off course. It's a moot point; with no manpower at the oars, we're not going anywhere – and we've got a long way to go.

It's 29 December 2022, and this has been the state of affairs for the last four and a half days. The reason for our situation? Steve and I have decided to tackle the Talisker Whisky Atlantic Challenge. Sadly, this doesn't involve drinking a boatload of whisky; rather, it's an attempt to row 3,000 nautical miles across the ocean. Seventeen days earlier, we set off from La Gomera in the Canary Islands, with the next time we experience dry land being when we land at the island of Antigua in the Caribbean.

Neither Steve nor I are strangers to pushing ourselves: we're both veterans of all manner of endurance events, from ultramarathons to triathlons, in a variety of the world's most challenging environments.

Neither of us have experienced anything like this, though.

When you're on land, you generally have the option of continuing to press on ahead. You might be dead on your feet, but every agonising step forward is one step closer to the finish line, and you're in control of those steps. In a situation like this, I'm entirely at the mercy of a very unpredictable ocean, and it's incredibly hard to deal with. Having competed in so many events where I had to keep putting one foot in front of the other for a seemingly indeterminate amount of time, it's deeply ironic that the hardest thing I've ever had to do is simply wait.

While I do exactly that, I've got a lot of time to think. The main thing I'm thinking of? Exactly how I got to this moment, with the Laurel & Hardy quote of 'well, that's another fine mess you've gotten me into' on repeat in my head as I look at Steve. I'm sitting in a cramped, sweat-filled cabin while I and my rowing mate of dubious musical talent wait to get on the oars – something that fills me with mixed emotions.

On one hand, we don't like this sitting around; we just want to get going again. On the other, it means going back to the grind. Back to the extreme tiredness; back to one-hour sleeping shifts; back to aches and pains and bruises and blisters in parts of the body that we didn't know were able to experience such sensations (and probably shouldn't).

In the meantime, it gives me a chance to reflect on the parallel journeys I've been on – both to take part in this race, and to where I am in life in general.

Chapter 1

Into the unknown

LOOKING BACK at the big moments in life, it's hard not to look for the germ of the idea – the moment or situation in which the journey began. For some it might be a moment of inspiration, while for others it's witnessing somebody do something similar, prompting the decision to ape their actions.

In my case, it all started with an email from my friend, Steve Hayes:

> Good morning Peter. Yes, that must be an official email as I used your full name.
>
> Amazingly I've been given the green light by Corina and work to row the Atlantic next year (2022/2023 Talisker Whisky Atlantic Challenge). I had planned to do this solo and fancied the challenge of doing it solo but part of me also wants to share the experience and I'd hate to do it solo if it's something you would like to do. It would be silly for me to do a row and then you do one the following year, it wouldn't make sense financially. A few bullet points below to give you something

to think about. Obviously the main concerns will be financial, as they are for me but let me know either way.

Have a think bud and let me know what your thoughts are. Test the water with Rach and the kids and give me a shout. If you have any questions let me know, I have tons of info.

Yours Sincerely,

Steve Hayes

How about it?

Steve was someone I'd got to know during my time both in Jersey and on the ultrarunning scene. We met in 2012 while I was training for the MDS. He was putting in the (aquatic) miles for an English Channel swim, and I went down to support him at one of his fundraising events (he later returned the favour at one of mine). We'd built up a bit of a friendship based on like-minded hobbies.

Steve is very much an 'all or nothing' type person, whether it's sea swimming in his speedos in winter, running around Jersey, or embarking on a heavy drinking session. I found him an enormously positive person to be around, and it's impossible not to have a laugh in his infectious company.

He messaged me quite a bit when I was out in the desert, with some funny messages to keep me going. One in particular made me laugh out loud when he pointed out that he was worse off than me, since his girlfriend had gone away for the weekend, and his 'downloading' plans had been adversely affected by his Wi-Fi going down on the same weekend.

When I got back from the MDS, I contacted one of my tent mates, Andy McDonald, who had performed exceptionally well out there. With this in mind, I quizzed him on how he had trained. He told me about this event called the OMM (Original Mountain Marathon), a two-day pairs event in the Brecon Beacons involving navigation and complete self-sufficiency. Steve agreed to join me, and we became mates from then on.

As you'll probably gather, having picked up this book and started turning its pages, I like a challenge. I've completed ultramarathons across desert, mountains, snow and jungle, traversed the length of an entire country on foot (admittedly it was Wales, but still), and pulled a car a marathon distance (a Smart car, but they weigh a fair amount; you try pulling one for 26 and a bit miles).

Still, rowing across an entire ocean – it's impossible not to feel more than a bit daunted by it; 3,000 nautical miles of almost unending blue – with depths of five miles at its deepest points – the majority of which comes without catching sight of another human, unless you're fortunate enough to encounter a yacht, passenger liner or cargo hauler (many of which are unmanned now, so don't expect any friendly waving from the deck). It can get a bit choppy, too – the waves have been known to reach as high as 30ft.

Then there's the issue of space: spending the entirety of your time on a boat not much bigger than a boardroom table, on which you have to store all your belongings, prepare all your food and perform all of nature's duties.

This is before we get to the physical exertion involved. Rowing as a pair, it could take anywhere between one and a half and two months. Having done a cursory bit of research, it seemed that most rowers in pairs went for the 'two hours on, two hours off' approach, meaning that sleep would be hard to come by – grabbed in snatches.

All this constant motion would have its consequences – weight loss being one. Even with a recommended daily calorie intake of 5,000 – around double that of the typical adult male going about his day-to-day life – you could still expect to lose potentially as much as three stone. A healthy rate of weight loss is generally a pound or two per week – obviously, this would far exceed that.

Finally, there was the rowing itself. While I'd done plenty of running and cycling, my actual experience of going out on a boat with a pair of oars was limited to the point of non-existence. 'Nautical novice' would probably be the most apt – not to mention accurate – description of me that you could come up with.

Not a lot of people had done it – visiting space and standing on the summit of Mount Everest are both feats that have been accomplished more frequently than rowing an ocean.

So, how about it? Absolutely.

Still, it wasn't as simple as deciding that I was 'up for it'. As much as people occasionally wistfully talk about getting away from all of life's pressures by sailing off into the distance, the actual reality of that was not quite so simple.

For a start, I have a wife, two children and three dogs. Rachel has shown an immeasurable amount of patience and understanding over the years and across the various challenges I've done – she even allowed herself to be dragged along on a few of them – but there was no getting away from the fact that this was asking a lot.

For a start, there was the massive amount of time I'd be away for. The longest I'd previously been absent was about a week – the two to three months that this would likely take massively dwarfed that.

Then there was the matter of work. Again, my employers had been incredibly supportive over the years, but I hadn't yet tested them by posing the prospect of having two months' worth of unpaid leave. An arrangement would have to be reached, and I'd have to plan ahead financially to ensure that everything was covered while I was away.

Finally, there was the challenge. Rowing the Atlantic is a big event, and safety is paramount, as you'd expect. To make ever such a slight understatement, there are significant risks associated with rowing an ocean, whether you do it as part of an organised race or outside of one (as recently as 2024, someone died while attempting to traverse the ocean, albeit not on this race). Atlantic Campaigns had an excellent reputation, and Steve and I decided that we owed it to our loved ones to do the challenge this way. We estimated the cost of taking it on could be anything from £120,000 to £140,000 – not a sum that either of us happened to have lying around in a shoebox somewhere. This would have to be funded through sponsorship.

Not to mention, all of this planning was taking place during the COVID-19 pandemic, and all the restrictions that entailed. While it seems like we're out on the other side now, nobody knew what the hell was going on at the time, or what kind of impact that would have on things.

While all of these seemed like pretty big hurdles, Steve and I consoled ourselves with the fact that Jersey is a relatively affluent jurisdiction, and we'd surely find someone to help us.

Even though I'd made up my mind that it was definitely something that I wanted to do, it wasn't something I approached the prospect of seriously, partly because I didn't truly think it would be possible. This attitude was partially influenced by the fact that I was a little bit in the doghouse with Rachel already – I'd recently finished an event, during which I ran the equivalent distance in miles on every day of the month – one mile on the first, two miles on the second, and so on. Considering the amount of time I spent away from home, not to mention the physical condition I was in (those of you who are mathematicians will note that I averaged marathon distance for the last 11 days of the month), I'd received quite the bollocking from Rachel: 'Peteloaf, you know I'm your number one fan, but what was so important about running over seven hours a day on your own when we could have been getting quality family time in?'

It was a valid point because the challenge was a bit pointless, and I'd taken things a step too far doing that. I ended up eating a fair amount of humble pie, and promised to be a bit more restrained in the future. So the timing of Steve's email perhaps wasn't the best!

There's no way I can do this, was my original thought. *This is something that someone else does.* Still, I mentioned it to Rachel anyway, framing it as, 'Guess what Steve's just sent me!' as she happened to walk into the front room.

Her response was instant – and completely unexpected, 'Do it,' she said. She sounded deadly serious.

More than a bit surprised at the positivity of her reaction, I inexplicably proceeded to almost talk her out of her approval of my own request.

'You're still annoyed with me about the last thing I did! Are you sure?'

She responded, 'That was a silly one; this one's more you; adventurous, an opportunity of a lifetime, and doing something with a good mate.'

I wasn't going to argue the case any further – I had her endorsement!

Further strengthening my faith in humanity to accede to my requests, work was incredibly supportive, too – they knew that this was something I was into, and the fact that I was giving them two years' notice.

'You utter madman,' was the response from my boss, Chris Clark, followed up by, 'Well, you are giving us two years' notice,' and followed up again by, 'How can we help you out with the challenge?'

The last comment sums up my employers perfectly – I've never known such a people-focused company. After that chat with Chris, I think I became a permanent addition to the risk register.

We knew that getting approval from work and family was the easy part, however. Along the way, we both had to learn new skills: becoming project managers, marketeers, finance people – we just had to become everything, as well as learning an entire new sport.

Without trying to come across as arrogant, both of us have been able to maintain challenging and rewarding careers – me in accountancy, Steve in hospitality – and, as such, we were adept at planning ahead. We quickly came up with a plan of action, the first part of which was to create a brand name for us to row under, reasoning that this would make it easier to market to prospective sponsors. 'Pete and Steve's insane rowing adventure', while evocative, probably isn't the most professional-sounding. 'Buoy-Zone' wasn't much better. After much spitballing, we settled on 'DragonFish' – the first part reflecting Steve's Welsh heritage, and the second nodding at my star sign, Pisces.

Having downloaded some previous competitors' sponsorship packs and looked at how they packaged themselves, we worked out a budget to provide a fairly accurate price for everything associated with the challenge, to include buying the boat. Once we had that, we had to work out how we were going to arrange the sponsors (i.e. Gold, Silver, Bronze), get branding designed for DragonFish, set up social media accounts, get a website up and running and recruit a support crew (to include physios, personal trainers and sports masseurs). Working together, this was duly achieved.

This was the first time we'd effectively project managed together, and we complemented each other. Every other Sunday evening, we'd let ourselves into my place of work, along with a couple of bottles, and work through our plan, assigning actions and setting deadlines. We took our respective deadlines seriously, and mutual trust was quickly cemented as we got used to a new way of working together.

I've always endeavoured to throw myself into things, and I applied the same mantra to rowing. This was essential – my only previous experience had been the occasional go on a gym rowing machine, or taking a rowing boat across the pond at my parents' old house (they had a lot of land). To this end, we visited the Jersey Rowing Club and got ourselves acquainted.

The rowing club has a few 'have a go row' sessions each year, aimed at beginners. We went down, introduced ourselves and announced what we had planned. Looking back, we could have forgiven them for laughing us out of there: 'Hi, we're here to learn how to row. On the subject, we're actually going to be rowing the Atlantic in two years. Can you help us please?'

As it turns out, our worries about experiencing a similar reaction as seen in the montage in *Cool Runnings*, where they unsuccessfully go around looking for sponsors, were very much unfounded. They were very accommodating and really supportive, with a notable mention going to Ian Blandin. A former Atlantic rower himself, he took us under his wing a bit.

Covid-induced restrictions meant that there were times when Steve and I couldn't row together, but Ian took us out solo and we learned that way. We spent a good year with the rowing club, during which time we became a regular fixture in the races in the pairs category. Despite competing against several people who had been doing this for far longer than we had, we actually did okay overall, and even had some silverware to show for our efforts come the end of the rowing season – not bad for complete beginners!

Keeping fit was something that we were accustomed to, but this was a new sport. In addition to joining the rowing club, we became very active in the gym, and also started one-to-one Pilates. A lot of this was new to me – whenever I'd gone to the gym previously, I'd mainly stuck to the treadmills, so going to the gym and getting a programme aimed at different muscle groups was something I actually found quite fun, as I enjoyed getting a bit of structure – the big change for me was doing Pilates. We got an amazing personal teacher called Sonja Assiter – she spent an hour with us a week, doing some pretty serious stretches aimed at flexibility and injury prevention. I'm not the most flexible of people, so I found this difficult at first, but stuck at it and enjoyed it. Our location was always a local park in St Helier at around 6.30am, so wind, rain or shine, we were there being put through our paces by Sonja.

The most important course of action, naturally, was to actually get hold of a boat. There were only so many ocean-rowing boats on the planet, and we needed one quickly and (relatively) cheaply. Some teams had bought them new, but this wasn't an option for us. Once the race was signed up for and the deposit paid, we started looking for a boat to purchase.

Thanks to a short-term loan from my dad, we were able to purchase one. An evening phone conversation along the lines of, 'Dad, I've decided to do that challenge that you didn't seem particularly keen about – how do you feel about lending me £20,000 for it so we can find a boat for sale?'

I explained that I anticipated it being a very short-term loan, since we were actively seeking sponsors. Dad was great, replying, 'Pete, no problem, although don't tell your mum, since I want no evidence I am associated with this.'

Meanwhile, Steve had been researching potential candidates, and duly identified a boat called *Sogno Atlantico*, which had just completed its fourth Atlantic crossing courtesy of a couple of French guys called Lilian and Guilhem. It had a good history, and we were encouraged to hear that it had never capsized (always a good characteristic in a boat). It was an Adkins Offshore rowing boat (not a Rannoch like most of the boats in the race), which meant that we'd be competing in the 'Open Class' category. It was about ten years old and looked its age on account of the general exterior condition and aged equipment, and was on the heavier side, but it complied with the rules.

One factor that complicated things was the fact that the boat was docked in Marseille. With both the UK and France still in lockdown, we couldn't go there to personally inspect it ourselves pre-purchase, so we had to take a bit of a leap of faith and get someone to collect it for us. Despite this, we were happy – just the knowledge that the boat had recently done the crossing and arrived back in one piece was enough for us.

Predictably, on arrival into Jersey, it was a bit of a mess, but this wasn't the worst part. Upon seeing the boat, my inner *Star Wars* geek took over. I said to Steve, 'This bucket of bolts is never going to get us across the Atlantic.'

Steve just smiled, rather than telling me a positive fact about the rowing equivalent of the Kessel Run.

There was a hole in the hull of the boat, which we strongly suspected was down to some questionable forklift driving during transit. We trusted the sellers, and knew the boat had left Marseille in good condition, so we were willing to give them the benefit of the doubt. Luckily, we managed to get the hole fixed very quickly by a fibreglass chap in Jersey.

The interior wasn't much better, for different reasons. The boat arrived almost exactly how Lilian and Guilhem had left it upon arrival in Antigua, so we had to empty everything and clean it from top to bottom. We also had to work out what equipment we could keep and what we'd need to throw out – this took a while, since neither of us were sailors, and didn't really know our way around a boat yet. This would all change.

We unveiled the boat at the Super League Triathlon – a very popular event in Jersey that brought a lot of people to the area. By this point, we had about half of the sponsors lined up – it was an opportunity for us to put stickers on the boat with 'Your logo here', to give an idea of what to expect if you chose to become a sponsor. While we didn't get a lot of interest on this front, it gained a fair bit of attention, as a lot of people hadn't seen this kind of boat before, so it was a useful weekend.

In terms of a name for the boat, officially we never changed this, as it's supposedly bad luck to do so (it was in our best interests to keep Poseidon on our side, after all), but we told our title sponsor that he could give it an official race name, which would be on the side of the boat. He chose 'Lilly Mae', the name of his granddaughter – a lovely gesture, I'm sure you'll all agree.

However, while we were at the Super League Triathlon, one of the visitors introduced herself: 'Hi, I'm the mum of Lilly Mae. By the way, you've spelled her name wrong.' Whoops! Not wanting to take the chance of misspelling the name of our own boat turning out to be bad luck too, we got it changed after that.

We also went to Teignmouth for one of the mandatory rowing courses, attended with a company called SeaSports Southwest. It was classroom-based for about a week – with the use of the pool for the survival part of the course – and we did it with about 20 other rowers, so it was fun to absorb all the knowledge associated with the challenge and ocean rowing in general, as well as brainstorming ideas with other teams. The days were quite full-on, but it was useful to immerse ourselves in the ocean-rowing world we'd joined for a whole week.

We attended alongside two other teams that would be competing in the same year's race as us: solo rower Mike Bates (aka The Atlantic Grappler), and the trio of Laura, Millie and Frankie (aka The Atlantic Girls). We all stayed in the same B&B for the week, and there were one or two boozy nights as we got to know each other a bit more. The girls were lovely – all close friends from university looking to achieve their dream together.

Mike, a seriously impressive and focused individual, was a Brazilian jiu-jitsu black belt and a former MI5 agent. He was deadly serious, but had a great sense of humour. I remember one of his quotes when he appeared on one of the daily recordings when we were out in La Gomera. It was something like, 'I'd like to say I rowed an ocean, rather than half an ocean or a quarter of an ocean.' He was of course referring to the challenge in relation to the team size, and when this was aired in front of the whole fleet, there were resounding boos in his direction. I remember glancing over and seeing him with his head in his hands.

The final day of the course was particularly useful, since this was a dedicated ocean-rowing day course facilitated and hosted by Ian Couch from Atlantic Campaigns. Ian has been a key figure in the race for years, and the day spent with him was invaluable. I came away with pages of notes and lists of actions.

Tim Cox was our teacher on this course, and Steve and I both formed an instant friendship with him – we knew he did weather routing for people, and asked if he'd do that on our race. Barry Hayes was recommended to us when it came to managing our social media while on the row, so we recruited him to do just that, and put aside some budget to get him on board. In hindsight, investing in Barry was one of the best decisions we made. He'd completed a couple of rows himself, and was a true ocean-rowing expert and amazing at Atlantic storytelling.

Things were falling into place, and we came back to Jersey feeling a lot more prepared, but there was still plenty more to do. Mike already had his boat in the water, and was streets ahead from where we currently were in respect of our plan, so I did feel a little daunted by this. Our number-one action on getting home was to get our ocean-rowing boat in the water, get some much-needed practical experience and commence our qualifying hours. The race was on.

Interlude 1.1

I FIRST met Pete while I was swimming in the Havre Des Pas Lido, a tidal swimming pool on the south coast of the island we'd both decided to call home: Jersey.

I was training for an English Channel swim, and in order to raise more money for charity and to get some decent training in, had decided to do a 24-mile/24-hour swim in the pool. Pete heard about this through a mutual friend and decided to come down to support me from the poolside, which I really appreciated. Not long after that swim, I heard that Pete was running on a treadmill in our local Marks & Spencer to raise money for his chosen charity prior to embarking on the Marathon des Sables. I popped in with my family to offer some encouragement and drum up some donations.

I didn't hear much from Pete for a while until he approached me about a race he was interested in, the OMM (Original Mountain Marathon). He'd heard about it, and needed a partner, as it's a pairs race. He asked if I'd be interested, to which the answer is usually yes. He needed to submit an application detailing our previous mountain experience. I emailed him setting out all the mountain ultramarathons I'd completed, and he came back promptly and suitably impressed, stating that he didn't realise I was so experienced. I confessed that I'd actually made them up, but said we'd be fine – I was an army cadet, after all!

We were accepted and started our planning. In that first weekend together, we travelled to Bristol via plane, hired a tiny little Smart car (as we both have a tendency to be rather frugal) and drove to the Brecon Beacons via a quick stop to see my mother. By the end of the weekend, we'd shared a very uncomfortable night in a Smart car, an even more uncomfortable night in a one-man tent on the side of a hill in a muddy field on Halloween weekend and then, to top it off, a night in a double bed at my sister's house. It was a very quick way of getting to know someone!

Following that first race, we entered our first 100-mile ultramarathon about four weeks later – the Winter 100 by Centurion. That included another long weekend together and 29 hours in the pain cave witnessing each other's highs and lows, moans and grumbles.

We ventured to Brazil for a couple of weeks in 2015 to take part in the Jungle Marathon. At 260km of dense Amazon jungle, it was far more than a marathon. We completed several other ultramarathons together in the UK and Romania, and got to know each other well.

When I decided that I'd like to row across the Atlantic, there was naturally only one person to invite along to share the experience. It had been on my bucket list for years, along with some other exciting adventures. When my wife suggested I start ticking them off, I didn't need to think for long, but I did want to share the journey with someone – and who better to ask?

Steve Hayes, friend, fellow ultramarathon runner
and rowing partner

Interlude 1.2

LATE ONE Sunday morning in 2009, I did something that most Londoners avoid, and that I've never done before or since: travel into the city on marathon day.

After hours of queues and wandering around on my own with no phone signal, I eventually managed to meet up with Pete at the end of the race. To most people, running a marathon is the end goal that they aim for after months of training. It didn't occur to me that for Pete it would be only the beginning.

I didn't even realise that there was something bigger than a marathon. After all, the word 'marathon' comes from an old Greek legend where the bloke who ran the distance died at the end of it.

It certainly didn't occur to me that, years later, he'd be showing me the two-person boat he was planning on using to row across the Atlantic Ocean, and making jokes about the dire fate that awaited the unfortunate buckets that would be accompanying him.

In the years since that first marathon, Pete has not just rowed across oceans and run ultramarathons but he has crossed the Sahara desert, the Arctic Circle and the Amazon rainforest.

After one ultramarathon in the snow where he had to get rescued, we laughed about a telling-off he got from

Dad, where he was told, 'For Christ's sake Pete, you have children.'

When I was a kid, I remember him having some weights in his room and playing a bit of football, but I wouldn't have guessed that he'd have got into all this. I've done my best to keep up: I tried to run 5km with Pete one Christmas, but started limping halfway round with a bad knee. That earned me the nickname 'unfit brother'.

On the morning after a day of heavy drinking, I wake up late feeling like death, while Pete wakes up early to run a marathon. I can't keep up with Pete, but I can make jokes about him. One that never grows old is asking, 'What are you running from?' each time I hear about his latest race. I'm hoping to discover the answer to that question in this book!

Alan Wright, Pete's brother

Chapter 2

From Dorset to Jersey and beyond

BIOGRAPHIES OF accomplished sportspeople seem to have a running theme: utmost dedication to their vocation of choice. This invariably involves them getting up at the crack of dawn every day from the age of six to practise their passion, reluctantly trooping off to school, then getting home, only to immediately go outside and carry on as they were before. Indoors is only revisited either when it's dark, or when they get dragged back in by their concerned parents.

That wasn't me.

In fairness, it's not like I was inactive. Growing up in the town of Poole in Dorset, I played a lot of football with friends – both kickabouts down the local park and for various five-a-side teams (sample team name: Borussia Bacardi – nope, they didn't supply us with any free alcohol for our efforts in promoting them).

Perhaps learning our lesson, we later managed to convince the landlord of our local pub to supply us with kit for one of our newly formed teams. In return, we'd name our team after his fine drinking establishment.

Admittedly, we may have stretched the truth a bit about our athletic prowess. Based on our initial boasts, he may have got the impression that we were some dedicated semi-professional outfit, rather than filling out the league at Poole Sports Centre. After our very first game we all paid a jovial visit to the pub and he excitedly brought the drinks over to hear all about the match.

'So lads, how did you get on?'

'Lost 9-0!'

The change in his facial expression was priceless.

Side note: despite the varied nature of all the events I've participated in over the years, and some of the potential dangers those entailed, my worst injury actually occurred during a game down the local park at the age of 17, where I managed to break my leg. Through on goal, the keeper came out with a rather nasty two-footed challenge that connected with my shin. The loud 'crack' my bone made as it fractured didn't seem enough evidence of serious injury to my friends, who laughed as I hopped off the pitch. The subsequent hospital visit confirmed that I wasn't play-acting!

The next eight weeks were spent with my leg in plaster. I never liked sitting still, so this time – even with the latest *Championship Manager* game on my Amiga to tide away the boredom – isn't something I recall fondly.

I played a fair amount of squash, too – again, never to a massively high standard, but it was a good workout, and satisfying to see myself rise up the rankings after a win. However, as much as I loved the game, the red mist would occasionally descend, and quite a few racquets were destroyed in the process.

Prior experience of running was thin on the ground – one memory stands out at an old school sports day, and entering a long-distance race. Minimal training later, my mild asthma meant that I suffered straight away, thus ensued a neck-and-neck with another kid, both of us miles behind in last place. Determined to avoid the dreaded wooden spoon, a sprint finish sealed my finish in second from last place. Perhaps this was a sign of some competitive spirit that would prove to be handy later on!

Speaking of asthma, this was something that played up a few times when I was younger, along with some quite nasty bouts of hay fever. I had a few attacks – one even saw a school trip coach being diverted to pick up some antibiotics from a local town.

While these were recurring issues for me when I was a child, ultimately they bothered me less and less over the years. I still carry an inhaler with me during every event I do, but to date I haven't needed it. It has become more of a good luck charm than anything else.

Interestingly, when Covid jab season came around, I was the only member of my family who was deemed to be 'high risk' – despite my mum being diabetic and having recently recovered from cancer, and my dad having high blood pressure!

Beyond that, my life went on a pretty typical trajectory – I studied hard, and got my GCSEs, followed by A-Levels. After a few months of studying the latter, the wonderfully encouraging teachers at my school helpfully predicted that I'd fail everything on the basis that I wasn't academically up to it. I've never enjoyed having limitations placed on me – particularly by those I have little respect for – so I resolved to pass all of them. This was achieved through putting in excess hours and seeking outside help for a subject I found particularly challenging – mathematics (despite being told that I was unlikely to get them – again).

On leaving school, I set my sights on becoming a trainee accountant – which was perhaps a surprising career choice, given the opinions of my teachers regarding my mathematical prowess! I saw this as an opportunity to obtain a degree-equivalent qualification, while also presenting me with good opportunities for the future. However, the UK was in the midst of a recession, so I had to settle for a job as a cashier in a high-street bank. This turned out to be a relatively short stint – from day one, in my spare time, I hand-wrote letters to every accountancy firm in the Yellow Pages in the hope of getting a job. After countless rejections, I was eventually offered a role as a trainee accountant in a small local practice. While I had to take a pay cut from £6,800 down to £6,000, I'd gained a foothold in accountancy. It's a career that I've carried on for much of my life, and generally found pretty fulfilling.

Outside of that, however, the rest of my life wasn't quite happening. I met someone in my early 20s, and we moved in together and got engaged. Looking back, we did this far too quickly. After a couple of years, I wasn't feeling entirely happy, and decided to end the relationship. However, outside pressures and a feeling of general confusion resulted in me going back and giving it another go, and we remained together for another couple of years.

During this time, I almost accepted my fate of being in a relationship I wasn't happy with, and the weight piled on. Ironically, the second and final time it ended, I was the one who got dumped, as she revealed that she'd met someone else. Rather than the sinking feeling you often get when a relationship ends, my chief emotion was of delight. It felt good.

The weight was still a problem, however. It got to the point where breathing in and holding in my stomach wasn't making much difference anymore. I remember being on a night out, and looking at my reflection, thinking, *Is this it, now?*

I was 28, and felt badly in need of a change.

Sometimes, fate intervenes in interesting ways. This came in the form of a surprise job offer. Someone I used to work with had asked if I was interested in working for his new company. Without a massive amount tying me to Dorset due to my recent break-up, I decided to give it a go. There was just one thing: not only would I be moving areas, I'd be moving to a different island entirely, and effectively starting all over again in a place where I knew just the one person. It turned out that this was exactly what I needed to set myself on an entirely different trajectory.

If you haven't visited Jersey, then it may come as a surprise to discover that it has a lot more going for it than you might imagine. Containing some incredible beaches and outdoor areas, and with a pretty vibrant social scene, it's an absolutely breathtaking place.

There's a lot of history to the area, too. As well as the various castles and burial sites, there are many reminders of the island's time during the Second World War. The Channel Islands were the only part of the British Empire to be occupied by Nazi Germany, with the end of this being commemorated every year on Liberation Day on 9 May.

All in all, there are definitely worse places to live.

Even so, I wasn't expecting my stay to be a long one. At that point in my life, I felt like I was in a bit of a rut, and just wanted to try something new. I didn't expect to be there for much longer than a year.

So, armed with a couple of suitcases and my cat, Austin, I set off on the ferry from Poole, pitching up at my rented flat near St Brelade's Bay, having let out my old place in Bournemouth (residency laws in Jersey mean that you can't buy a house until you've lived on the island for at least ten years).

The first year was a bit wobbly, and didn't make me fully convinced that I'd made the right decision. I didn't know anyone, and it didn't help that the guy who had got me the job abruptly left the company only a short time after I'd started. I was now very much on my own! Plus, I worked on an industrial estate outside town, so it wasn't exactly a great social hub – not ideal for getting to know people.

Regardless, I threw myself into island life, gradually built up a circle of friends and, with it, a social life. One of my first observations about Jersey was how generally active people were – perhaps more than anywhere else I've been, it seemed like there were always people out and about, surfing or paragliding, getting involved in rugby or football, or running along the seafront. This was where I first got the idea of taking on a marathon.

I initially tried to join a football club – more for the social side of things – but quickly realised that I wasn't really interested anymore. It all seemed to be taken a bit too seriously, and wasn't as much fun as it used to be when I was just having a kickaround with my mates. So I did a bit of running independently and later joined up with a couple of people I'd got to know. The runs were generally at a slow pace and involved me rocking up in my football socks and five-a-side trainers. I wasn't quite ready at this point to join a running club, and was fairly clueless when it came to things like kit.

Having caught the bug, I entered and completed the Great North Run – a half-marathon – as a tester, which I really enjoyed. The atmosphere was incredible; I'd never competed in anything like this. The thrill of being around other like-minded souls and constant encouragement from complete strangers was so uplifting. From then, I aspired to do the London Marathon.

Anyone who has tried to enter the London Marathon will know that simply applying usually isn't enough; it's consistently over-subscribed. The only way to guarantee a place is to enter on behalf of a charity, who usually require a large sum to be raised. Everyone else has to go through the lottery of the ballot, which I duly entered. Amazingly, I got in first time.

Despite having my entry confirmed, I still didn't really have the belief that I could actually do it. During my training, I picked up plenty of sore-shin-type injuries. My GP and friend, Dr Harris, could see how determined I was, but could also see what a complete cowboy my current physio was, so he recommended I see a new physio by the name of Lisa Mann.

I recall my first consultation with Lisa as I explained my background and the issues I'd been having since taking up running. After putting me through various tests, Lisa stated, 'Pete, you have very weak core strength.' She wasn't one to mince her words!

After further analysis and explanations, I was provided with a strength and conditioning plan to get me where I needed to be, while being encouraged to keep on running. This was a complete game-changer and I never looked back. I ended up working with Lisa on numerous events over the years, so it turned out to be a great recommendation.

Eventually, I rocked up in London with my wife, Rachel, and completed the marathon in 4 hours 14 minutes. It felt like job done.

Speaking of Rachel …

During this time, my life continued to change in ways I hadn't imagined it would when I first made the trip part-way across the channel. I met Rachel when I was interviewing her for a role at the company I worked for. First impressions were interesting and contrasting. I think it was love at first sight for me but, as it turns out, Rachel actually thought I was gay. This was apparently on account of me being very polished in my appearance. A couple of days after the interview, I decided to deliver the news via a phone call.

'Hi Rachel, this is Peter. I'm afraid to tell you that we've selected someone else for the role.'

'Oh.'

'Only joking, you've got it really, hahaha!'

From memory, Rach called me a bastard and then laughed. They do say women love men who can make them laugh, but I guess there are better ways of doing this!

After a year or so of flirting, we ended up together. We got married in Hawaii in 2006, and not long after, had our first child, Josh.

In terms of fitness, I fell back into playing the occasional game of squash and running 5km races here and there. Both Rach and I were in challenging jobs that we enjoyed, and outside of that we were taking on the new adventure of parenthood.

As any parents will know, it's all-consuming. Fitness took a back seat for a while, and I put on weight again, thanks largely to the sustained habit of comfort food and working long hours with minimal time away from the desk. In 2010, my second child, Leila, was born. My existing habits continued.

I realised that something had to change one day at work a year later, when I was forced to carve a new notch in my belt. It was around this time in the kitchen at work that I heard a radio shout-out looking for marathon runners to be part of a charity team for the London Marathon. Seeing my prohibitively bulging waistline as a sign, I put my name forward.

As it turned out, this one was a bit of a shocker for me. Having a better idea of what to expect this time around, I didn't do quite as much training as I had previously – or indeed, as I should have done. This was the first time I'd made this mistake, and it wouldn't be the last.

I rocked up in London a couple of nights before and decided to meet up with my good mate, Rich, on the Friday night. Having not seen him in a while, I made the most of a rare child-free night, and got well and truly hammered.

While the marathon was to take place on the Sunday, leaving me with a bit of time to nurse the hangover, I still felt pretty dehydrated come the starting line, and no way in optimal fitness. I was learning the hard way all the lessons that bad preparation can teach you – this manifested in me using a belt I hadn't worn before to contain all my running gels. Two miles in, this fell off, landing somewhere irretrievable. Bugger.

At mile six, bad preparation gave way to bad luck as I caught my foot on a divot, causing me to fall and twist my ankle badly. I resolved to run on adrenaline for as long as I could, and then come up with a plan B. To compound matters somewhat, I didn't have any snacks with me, forcing me instead to rely on some unfamiliar-looking gels that were being handed out by race-side volunteers. This was another mistake.

On the dietary front, one piece of advice that tends to be given to long-distance runners is to stick to what you know. Not doing this came back to haunt me, as one or more of these gels clearly had an unfavourable impact on my stomach.

It was getting better and better: first I had an ankle that was rapidly swelling, and now I was in desperate need of the toilet.

With no Portaloos in sight, I had to duck out of the course and nip across the road into a rather 'interesting'-looking pub, where I sat for ten minutes thinking, *What an absolute disaster. This is such a low point*, while doing what I needed to.

Still, despite these setbacks, I managed to get my head down and make it to the end in 4 hours 39 minutes – at no point did it cross my mind to quit. I learned the power of mental resolve that day. It was something that would serve me well in the coming years – and in all honesty, I probably got more out of this in terms of valuable lessons than I did the first marathon. That said, everyone else in the charity team seemed to have achieved a personal-best time. I was the exception in this, so I was a little bit out of sorts at the afterparty. It was another reason why I resolved to better prepare next time.

I wasn't immediately thinking about the next challenge, but sometimes life presents you with opportunities – or at least puts you in contact with people who plant those seeds in your mind. One such person was a really nice chap called Paul Burrows. A fellow Jersey resident, he also took part in the London Marathon as part of the team. We got to know each other during the build-up, and quickly became good friends – remaining so to this day.

Like I said, I didn't have any immediate plans on what was next, but Paul did. As it turns out, there was a race that he'd dreamed about entering, and managed to persuade me to join him. I actually never really believed I'd be accepted or meet the criteria, but I went along with it – why not? To my surprise – and horror – I managed to secure a place in the 2013 edition of the Marathon des Sables. If I thought the London Marathon was as bad as it got, I really was in for a rude awakening.

Interlude 2.1

GROWING UP together, lots of my memories of Pete are a bit vague – he was my annoying little brother, after all – but I do remember a shared fondness for certain TV programmes from the early 1980s that we would watch together – *Blake's 7*, *Monkey* and *Star Trek* being a few. When Dad's work took him to Japan in 1981, we as a family went with him. It was here that Pete and I discovered a new TV gem: the Japanese cartoon *Robots*. Pete, I believe, still has an unhealthy obsession with the robots, and has collected some figures that I think he's allowed to display in his office at home.

During our time in Japan, Dad also 'encouraged' Pete and me to write a diary of our time there and all the amazing places we visited. We did visit some amazing places but, looking back at our diaries, we seem to have been more obsessed with what we had for breakfast or lunch that day, rather than what Mount Fuji looked like up close.

On a surprise holiday to Disneyland in Los Angeles, Dad saw all the overconfident American kids swarming around the dressed-up Disney characters and thought he'd like such a photo of his two very socially awkward English children with them. The resulting photographic evidence shows some of the most fake, uncomfortable smiles on two children you'll ever see, while standing about 10m away from the Disney character in question! I think Pete re-created one of these photos when we revisited Disney on a family holiday in 2007.

Pete developed bronchitis during one early holiday to Cornwall, prompting its premature abandonment. Maybe having this illness as a child spurred him on to want to achieve more physically. Later, I'd hear through the family grapevine that he was going to be running through the Amazon rainforest (as you do), doing the Polar Circle Marathon, or possibly pulling a car around Jersey! In addition to these, there were lots of 'little' races – just the odd 50 to 100 miles here and there. I remember going to work, and my colleagues would ask me what mad challenge my brother would be doing this week, not believing me until I showed them Facebook photo evidence.

When I found out he was rowing the Atlantic, I think that this was the first time I was genuinely worried for his safety. During the time he was away, I was on edge every single day.

I'd also like to add that I saw far too much of my brother's – and Steve's – bottoms in the photos that he and Steve shared online, which collectively have probably scarred me for life!

As for what the future holds for Pete and his challenges? Well, he's not climbed Mount Everest or flown into space – yet!

Anna Sullivan, Pete's sister

Interlude 2.2

IT'S 10 December 2022, and I'm sitting in the reception of a hotel in Dorchester, waiting for a mate to surface from his pit so that we can shake off our hangovers by having a big fry-up. Checking the dates, I realise that Pete is due to start his Atlantic row. Fuck, was it today? A quick WhatsApp message to show my support:

> *Looks like the big row starts soon, so a couple of bits of advice ...*
>
> *1) Don't die. I quite fancy cycling in France next year and don't want to do it on my own. Beers in Rennes won't drink themselves.*
>
> *2) Assert authority in the boat ASAP. If you need to start eating each other, have dominance over Steve and eat him.*
>
> *Good luck you massive twat.*

No reply for over a week. Maybe he is dead. No, he's too stubborn for that!

For me, I think the madness of Pete's 'Point Break' activities started while doing our annual cycle trip in France in 2011 or 2012. Between Dinard and Dinan, Pete casually slipped into conversation that he'd signed up to do the Marathon des Sables in a couple of years' time. I'd heard of this – people died, it sounded horrible. Lunatic! But he nailed it.

And nailed multiple other crazy events, including (spoiler alert, he didn't die) the Atlantic row.

We've been mates since school. The *Brian Clough's Football Fortunes* sessions on his Commodore 64 (it used to 'crash' when Pete was losing) have long since evolved to nights in the pub. I was there when he broke his leg playing football (it wasn't me!), when he put his arse through the window of The Rising Sun (nothing to do with me again!) and when he fainted due to illness and the cold in our shared flat (that probably was something to do with me). If you asked me after finding him on the floor of our derelict kitchen whether Pete would go on to do any of these extreme events, then I'd have said absolutely no way.

We still catch up. We still do our cycle trips to France, we still do our nights in the pub. Each time, Pete will mention that he's off to do some sort of race or activity that defies comprehension, and each time I'll feel that same sense of incredible pride of being his friend.

Ceri Morgan, Pete's friend

Chapter 3

Rowing and setbacks

STEVE AND I returned from the course at Teignmouth late in February, feeling full of confidence and better prepared for what was up ahead. Even so, with departure day nine months away, there was a lot to do. We had to get cracking in a number of respects.

To start with, we had to get the boat in the water. At least 120 hours of rowing at sea had to be logged before the event – currently, our total stood at a big, fat zero. During our discussions with the other teams at Teignmouth, we were mildly horrified to discover that most of them already had their boats in the water – ours was still in storage in the local boat park in Jersey, getting branded with our sponsors' logos. Reality check duly given, catching up with them was our primary objective on returning.

On top of that, we had to maintain our intensive gym sessions to ensure that we were in top shape. We'd both been very disciplined while we were away, purchasing a week-long membership at a local gym – we even went there most mornings. However, we were certainly eating and drinking very well, courtesy of the local bakery and our newly acquired ocean-rowing friends. Rowing administration had been intense in the lead-up to our trip away, so we figured that we were entitled to some play time. This achieved, we resolved to get back to it once we returned home.

We were also already receiving regular nutrition advice from a local company called True Food, and in-body scans to monitor fat and muscle alongside it. I initially met with Paul Garrod, one of the company's directors, and he agreed to help with 12 months of nutrition support in respect of the Atlantic row.

After my first in-person chat with Paul, it was clear that we had a mutual love of anything endurance-based, and I knew that I was in safe hands. I completed an initial food diary based on my usual habits, and sent this to Paul for review. In response, he suggested some subtle changes that would complement the plan to increase weight in a healthy manner while boosting strength and reducing our chances of injury. We then monitored the results – as well as my fat levels – via an in-body scan, which we did on a fortnightly basis at his clinic.

One subtle change Paul suggested was to perhaps cut down on my units of alcohol (this was far easier for me to do when I wasn't in Steve's company). Steve and I were also convinced that we could positively influence the result of the in-body scans by going to the gym immediately before in an effort to get a really good scan on the day. I'm not sure if this ever worked – I suspect it didn't. Paul also cast an eye over our food pack plan for the anticipated days at sea, making several sensible invaluable suggestions. These included specific products to add variety, as well as high-calorie powder-based nutrition that we'd add to our drinking water. I found the time I spent with Paul extremely beneficial, and the transformation physically from the first day I began working with him until my departure to La Gomera was positive and noticeable.

A few weeks went by after our return to Jersey, during which the island seemed to be getting battered by high winds on a frequent basis. This was playing havoc with our plans to get the boat in the water. Courtesy of Ports of Jersey, we had a mooring for the boat secured, and were desperate to get her in. As it turned out, we weren't able to manage this until the end of March, thanks to a combination of the rare good weather windows rarely syncing with our time off work. In the meantime, we focused our energies on trying to secure as many sponsors as we could. We'd already obtained most of our main ones, so the majority of the branding space on the boat was effectively already reserved.

Embracing our creative muscles, we devised two plans: the '250 club' (this was a more realistic way for small businesses or individual supporters to get involved: for £250, we'd place a small, branded sticker of their company logo on the gunwale of the boat), and 'Feed a rower for a day' (pretty self-explanatory: people paid for our food for a day of their choice, and in return got a shout-out on social media). Both proved to be very successful: not costing a lot to do, they represented manageable ways for small businesses and individuals to be able to support us.

Eventually, the day of getting the boat in the water arrived. As it turned out, this would not be without drama or incident. We were operating on a tight budget, and in the early days of boat ownership, we'd been gifted a trailer to transport it on, which it had been stored in a boat park over the winter. Steve and I knew that the trailer had seen better days, but we were confident that it would be able to handle the short trip to the harbour. How wrong we were.

A good friend of ours, Dave Salter, offered to tow the boat on the day, and Steve and I followed closely behind in Steve's car. Around the halfway point, Steve's eyes narrowed, and he frowned.

'Is it just me, or is one of the back wheels wobbling?' Clearly, it wasn't just him, as sure enough, out of nowhere, the same wheel flew off, hit a wall and rebounded over the other side of the road. Thankfully, there were no other vehicles or any pedestrians around – facing trial for manslaughter via wobbly tyre might have hampered race preparations somewhat!

We sounded the horn at Dave for him to stop, and took a look. Despite the trailer now being a three-wheeler, we decided to embrace our inner Del Boy, take it slowly and complete the journey. The next ten minutes felt like an awful long time, with our eyes firmly fixed on the remaining wheels. Fortunately, this passed without further catastrophe, and on arrival the boat was swiftly placed in the water, upon which we rowed it to the mooring we'd secured. As for the trailer? It was swiftly – and fittingly – sold for scrap.

Now that the boat was finally in the water, we were able to start making inroads into the hallowed 120 hours. But even then, there were obstacles. One of the conditions was that Steve and I had to be in the boat together for them to count, which in itself presented a challenge when it came to staying out for longer periods of time, since our working hours and general availability were very different. However, for the shorter-distance rows, we settled into a routine of early mornings or early evenings, and were gradually able to start clocking up the hours. The purpose of these rows was not only to get used to being on the boat, but to practise using the equipment that we would come to rely on. As per the race rules, we were required to complete a log book in which we verified what we'd tested for each row.

The main issue we had with our training rows was that we were always faced with an 'out and back' route, which invariably meant rowing into the wind for one of the directions. It was here that we realised how difficult it was to control our heavy boat when rowing into headwind, or through crosswind. However, the training was good fun, and we were getting plenty of attention from locals who had never set eyes on an ocean-rowing boat before.

As part of our sponsorship and fundraising strategy, we were able to get the boat on display at the annual Jersey Boat Show. The day before the show, we rowed it the short distance to the neighbouring pier in preparation for the fact that we'd be there for two days. The show was excellent, and we managed to get plenty of exposure. We were also able to invite members of the public aboard to have a tour of the boat. It's safe to say that it captured everyone's imagination, and it certainly provided a boost to our fundraising efforts.

We were now into early June and had managed to accumulate a fair few training hours. However, these had all been two-to-three-hour rows – relatively brief in the grand scheme of things – so we decided that the time was right for a 12-hour overnight row, and booked one in. However, in the days before this was scheduled, my world was rocked.

A couple of months previously, Rachel had been for a few scans due to experiencing some headaches. She was fairly convinced that the issue was connected to her sinuses, and had also been seeing an ear, nose and throat specialist in the lead-up to the scans. So by all accounts, we'd both viewed this as fairly routine in terms of day-to-day health. Her visit to our GP to receive the results resulted in some very unexpected, and more serious news: she had two brain aneurysms.

The general way she was treated during this consultation left a lot to be desired, since she was basically given the news and shown the door, without any explanation of next steps or indication of whether the headaches were even linked to the aneurysms.

Rachel called me immediately after the consultation, and seemed calm enough.

'Hey babe. They've ruled out certain things, but it turns out I've got two brain aneurysms.'

Stunned silence followed. I knew she'd be running through scenarios in her head, and I wasn't fooled by the calmness in her voice.

Luckily, she wasn't one to sit idly by and accept this. The next day, she contacted the surgery and insisted on a follow-up appointment so that the next steps and treatment could be firmly understood. I did the same, making several rather forceful calls to the surgery.

We'd have to wait a couple of weeks before we knew what was going on – the uncertainty was very tough. Out of desperation, we did what the vast majority of people likely do when faced with this kind of news: start researching brain aneurysms on the internet. Unsurprisingly, online self-diagnosis didn't help.

Suddenly, the row didn't seem all that important anymore. I was fairly convinced that I wouldn't be doing it at all.

It's tricky to say much about the overnight row that we'd been planning for ages – it simply happened, without incident – not that anything would have stood out, as unsurprisingly my mind was on other things. I wasn't even thinking about the row, to be honest. I went out feeling pretty numb, and did the row with Steve pretty much just because we'd planned to do it – it felt a bit pointless, as I didn't really think that I'd be doing the row at that point. I needed assurances about the severity of my wife's condition.

I didn't really open up to Steve about how I was feeling, since I didn't have the answers myself about the situation. What could he say to make any difference? At this point I was just focused on helping Rach get through the weeks up to the date of the consultation, where we could get some clarity on the size and risk of the aneurysms.

The next few weeks were slow and tough. Rachel's headaches were intensifying, which she was convinced were linked to the aneurysms, and that her head was going to pop. The most probable reason for the headaches would – understandably – have been the anxiety, stress and worry, and we'd later be assured that the headaches were 100 per cent not linked to the aneurysms. Rachel was even making plans in the event of something catastrophic happening, which was heartbreaking.

The days slowly ticked by, and finally the day of the consultation came. We were ushered into a room to finally hear more about the diagnosis, and exactly what the next steps would be. The size and shape of the aneurysms had been analysed by several experts in London, so this part was reassuring, as we were no longer dealing with probability and guesswork. To our immeasurable relief, the results revealed that it wasn't as bad as first thought – one of the aneurysms was very tiny, and we were told that there was definitely nothing to worry about.

The other was on the small side, albeit an odd shape, and they did want to take more scans on this, but indicated that this would not be any time soon on account of the small size and low risk. However, we were pretty much told that there was nothing to worry about, and they were just going to monitor everything annually, which lifted our spirits a bit.

After leaving the medical centre, I gave her the biggest hug that I could muster and simply said, 'Well, that's the first positive news in a little while. I think a drink or three is in order. Love you, angel.' We headed to the local pub.

Over the next few weeks, we both got used to the diagnosis, and were comfortable with the next steps. Rachel was prescribed medication to help with the headaches, which were still occurring from time to time, and this did have a positive impact.

We had a heart-to-heart about the row, and Rachel wanted me to continue with the project. Once again, it was game on.

As Steve and I progressed through August, we were mindful that we still hadn't completed our 36-hour non-stop row – another condition of entering. Again, coordinating our working hours so we could practise was an issue. While my working life was more or less 9–5, Steve's job running a hotel saw him working at various hours, and he was in the midst of a crisis at work due to severe staff shortages, which sometimes saw him donning an apron and cooking breakfast for the guests.

Our mandatory rowing times had to be done together – solo rowing didn't count – so making it work was essential. We planned ahead and decided that it had to be done over the August bank holiday weekend. While this seemed to represent a good time to get this underway, things seemed to go wrong almost from the very moment we opened our eyes. For a start, the weather wasn't good. I had my doubts about going out in the conditions, but when we told a few people at the harbour what our plans were, no one made any attempt to talk us out of it. We took this as reassurance that everything would be fine. As it turned out, we were wrong.

At dusk, we took our usual route out. At this point, the conditions were certainly manageable.

'What were we worried about?' I said out loud, more for my own reassurance than anything else.

After crossing the bay, darkness started to fall, and we took a southerly direction. Trying to mimic race conditions as much as we could, we decided on rowing solo, while the other went in the cabin. After an hour each rowing, we both came to the same conclusion.

'The wind's too strong,' said Steve. 'It's pushing us away.'

'Agreed mate. We also have to factor in putting the brakes on.'

Mindful that we needed to be back in Jersey within a couple of days, we deployed the parachute anchor – effectively the boat's braking system (in terms of dealing with the wind, although you're still at the mercy of the underlying currents), and retreated to the cabin for the night. It was an uncomfortable evening, but we were also very reassured as to how the boat coped in the conditions, since we knew that we'd be facing much worse during the race itself. This gave us confidence.

At first light, we checked our charts and were staggered to find how far we'd drifted from Jersey.

'Jesus, I think we're close to being in French waters now,' exclaimed Steve. We duly retrieved the anchor to commence the very slow row back to Jersey. However, the strength of the wind was too great to make any progress, and we reluctantly redeployed the parachute anchor.

We had a chat, and took a good look at the advance weather forecast to get a clearer picture. Our mistake had clearly been not doing this from the outset. The long-range forecast effectively revealed that these winds would be with us for the next four or five days. We weren't in any distress, and had more than enough food and water to keep us going, but we both needed to get back to Jersey for work. Reluctantly, we took a joint decision to contact Jersey Ports and request a tow back from any passing vessel.

This passing vessel, as it turned out, was an RNLI lifeboat. They'd just finished a rescue, and were in the area. Conditions had become more lively by the time they arrived, and we were in communication via our handheld VHF, so we reassured them that we were okay, and they quickly decided on the best course of action.

'They want us to do what?' I shouted.

'They need to pull alongside, and we need to jump from our boat to theirs,' replied Steve. This looked far easier said than done, and there was little margin for error. With the conditions crazy in terms of wind and swell, there was fortunately other assistance at hand in the form of a Dutch container ship. Messages were triangulated, and they acted as a shield to the wind while the operation was completed. The RNLI receive many plaudits, and rightly so – the skills they performed as they came alongside us, allowing us to jump in, were commendable.

Once onboard, we were briefly checked over, but they could see that we were fine. We were both inspired as we watched them complete the rest of the operation, and then watched our tiny boat being towed back as it bounced around the waves. It was certainly a good structural test for it.

As we neared Albert Pier, Steve said, 'I can't fucking believe it. Mick has put us on Facebook.'

Mick is a great guy who volunteers at the rowing club, and he helped us immeasurably throughout the rowing project. He'd often take television reporters out on the club rib so they could get footage to accompany features on us. In this instance, as we entered the pier, we could see Mick mischievously stood there with his camcorder, filming the whole sorry incident. 'Any publicity is good publicity,' I attempted to reassure both Steve and myself.

What followed in the coming days was a very unflattering headline in the local newspaper, which read: 'DragonFish Row crew preparing for the Talisker Whisky Atlantic Challenge are rescued by RNLI after getting into difficulty off Jersey'.

The article on the website was followed by a series of sarcastic and judgemental comments from various people on social media. (One genius suggested we talk to people or read books about those who had previously rowed the Atlantic. Happy enough to dish out unwanted advice, he was less happy to take our sarcastic responses, thanking him and saying that we wish we'd thought of that, while also posting a link to our fundraising page.) We could probably appreciate how it looked – attempted Atlantic rowers come unstuck while still within sight of Jersey – but we just had to ignore the local headlines and get on with it.

In hindsight, this was probably the best training row we could have had.

We found ourselves in crap conditions that we had to live in for about 17 hours, getting bashed around all over the place, yet we handled ourselves pretty well, deployed the sea anchor a couple of times and basically practised everything we'd be doing on the actual row.

The boat never really felt like capsizing, and this gave us tremendous confidence. I'd also become very seasick (something I used to get when I was younger, and hoped I'd grown out of), and resolved to find some more effective medication. Without this experience, I dread to think how bad it would have been during the row itself. While we were planning a capsizing simulation, and never got to experience that, being able to do a training row in less than ideal conditions was quite valuable.

Even so, there was still a sense of frustration. We hadn't completed the mandatory 36-hour row, so we were back to square one on that front, and running out of time. Ultimately, we completed it fairly close to the deadline in flat, calm conditions on the day of the Queen's funeral. We took no risks this time, and didn't venture far from Jersey.

Away from the rowing, things were sizing up. We managed to secure all our sponsors to include 250 clubs, as well as the 'Feed a rower' initiative. With all qualifying hours logged and evidenced, the boat was now back out of the water and on its brand-new trailer (with wheels that were firmly attached this time) at the local boat park. It was fully branded with our sponsors' logos and packed with all of our supplies and equipment.

Before long, it would be making its way across an even longer stretch of water.

Interlude 3.1

EVERYONE HAS their own reasons for choosing to row across an ocean. Most are either running towards or away from something, and the lure of the power and majesty of the ocean combined with the magnitude of such a campaign is sufficient for most to find whatever answers they might be searching for.

For me, it was to pay back the personal debt that I felt that I owed the doctors, nurses and facilities at Leeds General Infirmary who combined forces to save my youngest son's life. That, and to deal with the decade-long trauma I endured following that experience.

I first met Team DragonFish during our mandatory shore-based courses in Teignmouth, Devon. The humour and fun both Pete and Steve brought to what can often be quite dry topics of tidal streams and the colour and shape of cardinal marker buoys was a welcome relief. Their preparation was different, too.

We were sharing a house for the week with a number of other ocean-rowing teams. The house was situated a short walk from the training centre and, while we had our own rooms, we shared a communal kitchen and dining area. I never went to university but it's the kind of place I imagine (fairly affluent) students might share. It was definitely a step up from the military accommodation I'd been used to during my formative years. I was at the training course on my own, as I was to row across the ocean as a solo rower. Pete and Steve kindly adopted me, and we became good mates.

The first night, we all headed down to the nearest supermarket to stock up on supplies. As budding endurance athletes, we'd each recced the nearest gym and running routes and were, or so I thought, set for an intensive week-long training camp, both physically and mentally. It was upon returning to our accommodation that I realised that not all teams prepare the same.

I unpacked my Greek yoghurt, oats and protein bars into the fridge alongside one of the female crews, who too had purchased lean meats, salads, rice and bottled water. It was then that Pete and Steve entered the kitchen and started unpacking their own supplies: one extremely large bottle of single malt whisky, half a dozen bottles of red wine and a crate of ale. Now, before you get the wrong idea and worry that Team DragonFish hadn't considered their nutrition and macros carefully enough, they also pulled out a family multipack of crisps and assorted salty snacks. These two were athletes on a whole other level!

What impressed me the most about Pete and Steve during the first week that I got to know them both was not only how much they both could drink each evening, but the fact that they never missed an early morning gym session or were late to the training centre once – even after Steve broke a few ribs falling down a flight of stairs in the middle of the night, having polished off the whisky.

Their good humour and unique preparation followed them to La Gomera and the start of the race. They both lightened the mood of the fleet with their great humour and reassuring and well-founded confidence. They kept our feet on the ground leading up to race start, and for that I was extremely grateful.

Everyone has their own reason for rowing an ocean and their own way of preparing for that challenge of a lifetime. Pete and Steve showed that you can both prepare properly on and off the water and enjoy the journey at the same time.

Cheers to you both for that.

Mike Bates, The Atlantic Grappler,
fellow competitor

Interlude 3.2

I'VE KNOWN Pete in various capacities for around ten years or so, crossing paths at lots of social gatherings through our mutual friend, Steve Hayes.

Having trained Steve for a number of his events and races, I was asked if I could help both of them with the preparation for their Atlantic row (which was around 14 months away at the time of asking). We made a plan and cracked on with it.

It was clear from the offset that there were things Pete would do because he enjoyed them and things that he'd avoid because he didn't (even if they might have been in his best interests). If I'd asked him to run through a brick wall or move an object 100 times on repeat for 20 minutes, it would absolutely get done. Ask him to do some stretching and mobility work, and his eyes would glaze over (more on that to follow). Ask him to do that at home to supplement what we were doing ... nope. Hence my gym name for him being 'Captain Cardboard'. But we are getting there – he can now almost bend over and touch his toes without fear of snapping.

Since the Atlantic row, Pete and I have continued to work closely together, and I'm honoured to have played a miniscule role in helping him stay as strong and injury-free as possible. There have been numerous 100-milers here and there, and even more exciting things to come – some of it hare-brained, but if anyone is going to do it, Pete certainly is.

I was surprised when Pete mentioned he was going to be writing a book, but with so much experience and insight to pass on, I'm sure that there will be people out there who have much to gain from reading it. I say 'surprised', given that our exchange went along the lines of:

Pete: Yeah, so I'm putting some things together to write my book, finally.

Me: Mate, that's great. I'll have to have a think and come up with some anecdotes.

Pete: (That glazed look again). Yeah, that'd be great.

The following week, Pete turned up to his session as usual, but was at least honest in that he had no idea what an 'anecdote' was, and had to look it up in a dictionary.

Andy Glover, managing director, Sports Bug,
Pete's personal trainer

Chapter 4

Enter sandman

THE MARATHON des Sables (or the MDS, in shorthand) has long been a fixture in the ultrarunning calendar, and for good reason. If you're an ultrarunner, then as well as being more than a bit bonkers, you'll almost certainly like a challenge. The MDS duly provides.

Taking place on a 160-mile course across seven days in the Sahara desert, the hazards are numerous. First, there's the heat, with temperatures reaching as high as 50°C. Chugging water can only get you so far when you're rapidly losing valuable body salts.

Secondly, there's the relative isolation and unforgiving terrain. Over such a large distance, there are times when you won't see another living soul for quite a while. The race's creator, Patrick Bauer, conceived the event after wandering for over 200 miles across the desert without encountering any inhabited communities. While it's not quite as barren as his experience – the checkpoints staffed by volunteers make it a tad less daunting – there are certainly no crowds cheering you on.

Finally, there's the distance. A marathon is a challenge – try running six of them consecutively, in the heat and sand, while carrying all your gear on your back. Plodding along at your own pace isn't an option, either – there are cut-off times to adhere to, and stages that must be reached by a certain time limit. Fail to do this, and you're out of the race. All that preparation, all that money spent getting you there in the first place – it will all be for nothing.

Despite these hurdles – or probably because of them, in truth – the MDS is an incredibly popular race. Having begun life in 1986 with just 23 entrants, today well over 1,000 tackle it every year. Many ultrarunners choose the race to be their first overseas experience of ultrarunning – it's an iconic race, and regarded as a badge of honour to compete in it. Dubbed 'the toughest footrace on Earth', several books have been written about it, and various individuals renowned for not being averse to taking on a challenge or two have had a go (James Cracknell and Sir Ranulph Fiennes, to namedrop a couple). I'd now be attempting to join their number.

I'll rewind a bit. 'Bloody hell. How did that happen?' were my words to Paul when I realised that our applications had been confirmed for the 2013 edition of the race. I was convinced that I'd need far more on my running CV to actually be accepted. Paul chuckled and assured me that we'd both be more than capable of completing it. Once my place in the race was confirmed, I realised that I had a big challenge ahead. Despite the excitement, I also couldn't help feeling overwhelmed and apprehensive.

What on earth had I signed up for? Running through the desert? At least with the London Marathon you have the option of bailing out and going to the pub. There aren't any pubs in the Sahara that I know of.

Paul was less concerned. A far better runner than me, he had already completed a couple of UK-based ultras. On the flip side, I had my two London Marathon finishes, and not a lot else. Imposter syndrome was making its presence well and truly felt.

Determined to learn the lessons from my chaotic second marathon, I decided to have a go at my first-ever multiday event by way of preparation. Known as the Jurassic Coast Challenge, this effectively consists of three marathons taking place over three consecutive days along Dorset's Jurassic Coast (not far from where I grew up). This was decidedly beginner-friendly, with no criteria to enter, and the cut-off times were fairly generous. I didn't really consider myself an ultrarunner for the simple fact that I only had two London Marathons and a Great North Run under my belt at this point, so I didn't exactly throw caution to the wind on the first couple of days. I'm not sure why, but I guess I didn't consider myself ready, and figured that I'd injure myself if I pushed it too much. However, on day three, and with the encouragement of my good mate Stuart Glenister, who kept me company for that day, I pushed hard and finished the race strongly in a time of around five and a half hours.

There were a couple of invaluable takeaways from this race: firstly, I actually started to believe that I could tackle the MDS. Secondly, I met a man called Rory Coleman at the event. I first encountered Rory in the briefing tent prior to the race, and was very aware that he was a legend on the MDS circuit. I instantly warmed to him on account of his approachability, humility and great sense of humour.

His story was an inspirational one, and really resonated with me. One New Year's Eve, fed up with his bulging waistline and status as a hardened drinker and heavy smoker, he resolved to change his life. Unlike many who make these kinds of vows, he stuck to it, and then some. Three months later, having already lost three stone, he ran his first half-marathon. By the end of the year, he'd completed his first full marathon. Today, he's a veteran of over 1,000 marathons, and the conqueror of all manner of challenge events (one that stands out is a treadmill challenge that would see him attempt to break no less than nine Guinness World Records). If anyone could make an ultrarunner out of me, it was him. I decided that I wanted him to coach me. This would prove to be a very good decision indeed.

Once I'd signed up with Rory, I travelled to Cardiff to spend a couple of days with him. He made me feel right at home, and I felt at complete ease in his company – like I'd known him for years. He'd coached many novices like me, and I think he knew that my confidence needed building up.

We went to the gym for fitness tests and to set up a strength programme. Here, I was able to pick his brains about the race. We also spent a lot of time running through the admin associated with the race, and Rory emphasised the importance of making the right kit choices and keeping the race pack as light as possible. He'd seen so many people take 'just in case' items that they'd never really need, and would ultimately count against them due to the fatigue of carrying them for the entire distance of the race. He also gave me a great recommendation about sending my gaiters off to a haberdashery so they could be stitched on to my trail runners. This was an effective means of keeping the sand out throughout the race.

He also took me for an 'MDS pace' marathon with a suitable pack on. The whole weekend was invaluable, and Rory recommended a few good races that I should enter. The first was the Greensand Marathon, which was an out and back cross-country in Dorking. Rory had entered, too, and, desperate to impress him, I did the first half way too quick. I saw Rory around about the halfway point – he looked like he'd barely broken out into a stride. I clearly didn't.

'You've got your pacing all wrong,' he cried out. 'Slow it down.' In our earlier training sessions, Rory had emphasised the importance of consistency and finding your MDS pace that you could sustain. I duly 'blew up' on the return leg to the finish – a harsh lesson; I got overtaken by many runners.

Other recommended races included the Druid's Challenge (three days and 85 miles along Ridgeway in November), and the Pilgrim's Challenge (two days and 66 miles along the North Downs Way in February). They were both multiday ultramarathons and would involve basic accommodation (i.e. sleeping bags in a communal hall) on each night. It was the first of these (Druid's) where I met Sally Camm, Tom Carey, Gordon Marshall, Guy Pitcher and Joey Sharma, who were to be my future tent mates at the MDS. I really enjoyed Druid's, and felt stronger as the event went on. It was all coming together.

In between these two races – again on Rory's recommendation – I took on a race called Country to Capital, a 45-mile run from Wendover to Paddington. The idea was to get experience of the 'long day' at the MDS, which was a similar distance.

By this point I was in great shape, and felt very consistent in the first half. As mile 35 approached, I could see Sally in the distance, and made it my mission to catch up with her. Once I'd achieved this, we ran side by side for quite a while, chatting about anything and everything. However, as time went by, we wondered why we hadn't seen the left-hand turn to Paddington. Confused, we stopped at a pub and asked a local for directions.

'Five miles that way,' he said, pointing in the direction we'd just come. Damn. A 45-mile ultra had now become a 55-mile ultra, which still needed to get done within the race cut-off. At the first checkpoint after the turn to Paddington, I was told that I'd missed this, but I explained what had happened, and said I was confident I could make up the time.

'How about, if I do the next six miles in an hour, I can continue at the next checkpoint?' I suggested. A bargain was struck. This negotiation strategy was reused at subsequent checkpoints, and I finished the race with minutes to spare in second from last place. Regardless, I felt great. This was a massive confidence boost, and I was pleased with my bonus mileage.

Another useful training weekend was spent in Wales with Rory and around ten other MDS entrants. On day one, we trained on the sand dunes of Merthyr Mawr, and on the second day, we completed a couple of ascents of Pen y Fan – the highest peak in South Wales. In between all of this, we socialised and had ample opportunity to quiz Rory on everything MDS. There were absolutely loads of valuable insights here, and everyone was chipping in with questions about kit, nutrition, training methods and anything else that sprung to mind. I'd already heavily researched kit, but all of this gave me food for thought in terms of nutrition and all the testing I'd need to do in order to see what worked for me.

It was on this training weekend that I met Andy McDonald. Andy was a similar age to me, and more experienced in terms of running, having done events like the OMM and LAM, which had all been off-road and required good self-sufficiency and navigation. He and I hit it off straight away, sharing a similar sense of humour and a general determination not to become fat middle-aged men on account of our similar love of frothy ales and red wine. We'd have a laugh that we'd put everything into getting in shape for an event and then 'eat and drink like sailors on shore leave' post-event. It was almost the Ricky Hatton approach to recovering post-marathons. Andy would also be a tent mate at the MDS, and we'd go on to tackle quite a few events together.

The reaction of family and friends to my entry to the MDS was contrasting. Rachel was, as ever, my biggest cheerleader, probably having more confidence in me than I had myself. My dad's reaction was priceless. I told him over the phone, to which he solemnly responded, 'You don't have to do this son. You've got nothing to prove.' I think he'd read and believed the mythical account of the guy who got lost while running the MDS and survived on bat blood.

My close friends felt that this was a very 'non-Pete' thing to do, given that I was not exactly renowned for my athletic prowess. At this time, I wasn't exactly socialising with other long-distance runners, while Paul was looking lean and mean, and busting out some cracking distance times. I think I was viewed as the 'other local guy' going out to the MDS, with little surprise being shown if I returned with my tail between my legs. However, I had a quiet determination about my overall approach in the lead-up to the event, and I'd very much put myself out there in all the training events I'd done. This was going to be about running my own race, and looking to stay consistent and strong.

Finally, it was time to travel to the starting line! Taking a chartered flight on Thursday, 4 April 2013 from Gatwick to the city of Ouarzazate in Morocco, which, unsurprisingly, happened to be filled almost entirely with entrants for the race, was quite an experience. It was my first time in Morocco, but we didn't have any opportunity to explore on account of a late arrival time. Everyone had their own experiences and their reasons for entering – hearing them all really hammered home the level of the challenge I'd taken on. Everyone I spoke with had already done some big-ticket ultras. What had I done?

It was here that I met Richard Lendon, who had just completed the Spine race, a self-sufficient 250-mile race from Edale to Kirk Yetholm in the height of British winter. I was also sat behind Tobias Mews on the coach. A veteran of numerous events, I could hear him chatting to the person next to him, literally reeling off his previous experience, making me feel vastly inferior.

A comfortable night in a hotel in Ouarzazate was followed by a long day of coach travel to the desert – and our base camp. The journey was a long one, and we took a few comfort stops. At each stop, the temperature rose, it became hotter, and the terrain more unforgiving and dry. Civilisation was rapidly being left far behind.

The first night in camp was a very uncomfortable one: it felt like I'd had very little sleep. However, upon chatting to my tent mates the next morning, it turns out that I'd got more rest than I realised.

'Not sure how you missed it, but the bivouac collapsed during the night,' someone said. 'You just slept right through it.'

Saturday was admin day, which essentially meant kissing goodbye to our suitcases and having our kit thoroughly checked by the race organisers. All we had left post-inspection was our food, medicine and sleeping gear – all of which we'd be carrying with us for the week. This was probably a good thing – on the way over, I'd been constantly rummaging through my race pack, taking out bits and putting things back, so it was a relief to get rid of it and put a stop to any indecision.

One final call I made was to remove my inflatable sleeping mat, and simply rely on the thin layer of foam that made up the spine of my OMM 20L pack.

Come the next morning – and with it, race day – the previous day's decisions came back to haunt me. I'd had a very uncomfortable night on my thin layer of foam; I felt every little dagger-like stone that lay beneath me. Wake-up time was 5.30am – just as well, as I'd barely slept on my crappy thin foam bed. At 6am, it was customary for the burkas to tear the bivouac down. This, they seemed to very much enjoy, and it was done without warning. It didn't matter whether you were cooking or starkers; it came down. More than a few people found themselves in the latter category by the end of the race!

Despite the sense of nervous anticipation around me, I felt good, albeit mindful of the increasing heat and the load I was carrying on my back. At 12kg, the pack was heavier than I'd planned. Despite losing the sleeping mat, I probably still had far too many non-essential 'just in case' items. Rory had warned me about this, but there was no going back now.

The 7.30am briefing was followed by a rousing speech from Patrick – even after all these years, he was still enthusiastic about the race and its entrants. A born showman, he got us all very geed up as he switched between English and French, while encouraging us to jump and wave at the overhead drone. His passion was definitely contagious, and gave us all the extra push we needed. With that, at 8.30am – aptly to the blaring of AC/DC's 'Highway to Hell' out of the loudspeakers – we set off!

The first 12km felt just like my first marathon – I almost ran in a haze, not really thinking of any kind of plan, just not believing that I was really here in the middle of the desert, finally doing this after all the build-up. Soon enough, though, reality set in, and inevitably things started to get more tricky.

Relative to the rest of the course, the first day is designed to 'ease' you in (ha!), with a variety of surfaces: sandy and stony terrain, a few climbs, some small dunes and some seemingly never-ending plains. So nothing too extreme, in other words.

When you tell people that you're about to do an ultramarathon in the desert, one of the first things they tend to say is something along the lines of, 'Won't it be too hot to run in that?' From my experience, however, the most obvious issues don't turn out to be the biggest challenges – you spend so long agonising about them that, when it comes down to it, it's not as fearsome as the monster you've built up inside your head. And so it proved with the heat; it wasn't a huge issue. It was hot, sure, but I could hardly claim that it took me by surprise.

The flip side of this equation is that the things you never considered worrying so much about previously turn out to be an unexpected and unwelcome hassle – in this case, it was my rucksack. By the 20km mark, my shoulders were in a whole world of pain, which didn't subside for the rest of the course.

The rest of the day proceeded almost in a blur of excitement and pain, and the finish line for the end of day one came as a massive relief. Even so, past actions came back to haunt me. As I previously mentioned, you're not just losing water when you sweat; valuable body salts are dispensed with, too. To remedy this, it's recommended that you take numerous salt tablets throughout the day. In all the excitement, I'd forgotten to take my recommended dose, cue severe headaches. Lesson learned.

Meanwhile, the rest of the evening was spent cooking, chilling out and generally exchanging banter, which proved to be the typical post-race day evening. Andy, being the quickest, was generally the first in, so we'd all be giving him light-hearted grief on account of the abundance of stones under our makeshift mattresses. We advised him that, as first in, it was his job to suitably prepare the accommodation for the rest of us.

Darkness descended at about 8pm, signalling that it was time for bed. Unsurprisingly, sleep came to me a bit more easily this night, even though I still seemed to wake up every half hour. There wasn't too much snoring either, which was welcome.

The subsequent mornings generally followed the same theme. The bivouacs were pulled down at a very early hour to leave us to get ready for the day's racing on a rug, with sand swirling around us. My tent mate Tom and I would always have a pre-race day hug and wish each other good speed: 'Right, you sexy bastard. Let's get this done,' were the usual words before we hugged it out.

Tom was the life and soul of the tent, and the cause of much laughter for all of us. I recall once, when another competitor of elite standard visited our tent and made a rather critical comment about the size and style of Tom's race pack, Tom hadn't heard, but we told him after he left. 'The cheeky little bastard said what?' were Tom's words as he smirked. The light-hearted insults about the guy continued well after this race day, much to our amusement.

It was time for day two – mountain day! The centrepiece of this would be the climbing of three 'jebels' (local terminology for a hill or mountain). The jebels were, somewhat conveniently, positioned in order of toughness, saving the worst for last. Getting underway at 8.30am, it was noticeably hotter, with not a cloud in the sky. While the terrain was mixed again, it was to prove to be a much tougher day.

Generally, I'm a fan of climbing – I've always been more about the long-distance challenge rather than sprinting on ahead, so the slow attrition suits me just fine. In the event, the first jebel was conquered with relative ease. The second was a much more fearsome proposition. With the heat now at 40°C, by the end of that obstacle I could feel two hot spots on each heel: blisters. An inevitable occurrence, I was told, but still not what you want.

I reached the day's final checkpoint utterly exhausted – usually in a race, this would mark the point where the end is nearly in sight. If that was the case here, the view was blocked by a massive jebel – a sight that brought tears to my eyes. Quickly sorting out my fluids, salts and snacks in preparation for the onslaught up ahead, I grimly shuffled on.

The climb was as expected: relentless. In fact, I was later to find out that this jebel claimed a fair few of the race's withdrawals. Slowly but surely, moving on up in single file, the other racers and I eventually reached the top, after which we began our descent. As if to ensure we didn't finish the day by easing off, the MDS gods saw fit to grace us with a route littered by sharp rocks (my newly acquired blisters spitefully throbbed by way of complaint) and some lovely, tough dunes.

With that, day two was done but I definitely wasn't feeling confident. This stage had taken a lot out of me. With the knowledge that day four would be only a few miles short of a double marathon day (and there was still a whole day before I got to that!), I reappraised my approach, deciding that I'd slow down a bit and play it tactically.

In the meantime, I went back to the tent to recharge and go about my routine. Paul and Andy were already there, both looking far fresher than I felt. Their attitudes collectively backed up my push to pull myself together. 'It would be boring if it didn't hurt, Pete,' said Andy.

First up, though, was a visit to the medical tent, affectionately known as 'Doc Trotters', to get my heel blisters lanced. I didn't expect the screaming I could hear radiating from the tent as I queued outside to feel reassuring, but somehow it did; some blisters were clearly getting eradicated in there.

While I was getting used to camp life, I was really missing Rach and the kids. The messages we all received from friends and family on a daily basis really helped, proving to be inspiring for us all, knowing that people were tracking our progress and willing us on. It made me all the more determined to get this done.

Day three started for me at a relatively quick pace – so much for all my talk of taking it slowly! At the first checkpoint, I bumped into my tent mate, Sally, and I decided that it would be nice to share the day with someone.

Sally is one of life's lovely people, and she carries an abundance of positive energy as well as a permanent smile. She has a good role in marketing in day-to-day life, and manages a large team. It was clear to me why she was so good at this, given what a people person she was. I therefore spent the rest of the day walking and running with her. This was exactly what I needed: slowing things down, while giving myself a chance to recharge. Above all else, it was nice to have the company; it helped my state of mind no end.

The terrain was mixed – similar to the first day, although the temperature had dropped, which helped. It wasn't all clear sailing; the vast, flat plains never seemed to end, but the day went by relatively smoothly. It felt slower than my previous two, but I felt physically and mentally refreshed, and very much looking forward to the next day. As always, a nice cup of Sultan tea – a local favourite in Morocco – awaited at the day's finish line. By this point, the tent was feeling like a close family. The evening was a typically relaxed one, albeit foreshadowed by the knowledge that it would be the big one tomorrow: 75.7km in one day.

Day four – the one that would make or break me. It was a similar distance to the route around Jersey, which I've traversed on several occasions. Being mindful of the distance involved, I knew that I needed a consistent strategy. My plan was as follows:

1. Only run at the evening stage – before that would be strictly power-walking only.

2. Charge up my iPod, and pack it with motivational tunes to be used at various points in the stage. My main fall-back was the *Rocky IV* soundtrack, particularly the training montage. I found that particularly good when climbing things.

3. Get it done before midnight that day. Race rules allowed for around 30 hours to complete this stage, but I wanted to get it done within half of that time and, in theory, have the whole of the next day on camp recovering and recharging.

Pretty foolproof, right?

Since I started out at walking pace, it was no surprise that people quickly overtook me. On another occasion this might have been a blow to morale, but I kept plugging away, having confidence in my pacing and overall strategy. Sure enough, by the first checkpoint, this situation had reversed. While I was feeling confident, my optimism was quickly sapped by the growing heat.

By 11am, it had reached 54°C. I felt like I was being cooked alive – having been slightly blasé about the heat, now it became an issue. All I could do was plough on, working on getting the miles in the bank. My focus now was to be moving forward at all times while ensuring that I remained on top of my hydration and food.

By 3pm, as I marched across the vast sand dunes, the situation wasn't any better. It's at times like this that you rely on the banter with your racemates to keep you going, which I had in the form of Rory. A ten-time MDS veteran, his encouragement and knowhow helped keep me going. It was good being with Rory, and he was fast-hiking like me. At this stage, and having dealt with the severe heat, I felt pretty confident, and the fact I was moving as well as Rory meant I was doing something right.

While the temperature gradually dropped and my body heat level returned to normal, I started to feel more upbeat. At the fifth checkpoint – around the 60km mark – I bumped into a guy called Ian, and we chatted until the sixth and final checkpoint, generally about our respective drivers for doing this event.

Ian was a doctor in London, and we had a good chat about our backgrounds, families, reasons for the MDS and our bucket list. Ian had recently lost a loved one, and was very much doing this to honour their memory. Time flew, and again the simple act of a conversation with a like-minded soul really fuelled my positivity. From here, I felt like I could run until the end. I just about managed it.

I rocked up at the finish line at 11pm – I'd been going for 14 and a half hours. The reassuring cup of Sultan tea was followed up by an equally comforting hug from Tom Mullen, our MDS race rep. Tom was a young chap and part of the MDS team, and we'd seen quite a lot of him from arrival in Morocco. He'd always be there to see us in, and would encourage us to perform a little routine in front of the webcam on completion of each stage.

While this was all very welcome from a morale standpoint, physically I was in pieces. My right foot was ablaze with blisters, one on each toe. Thankfully, the next day was a rest day so I had time to recover. Even so, the night was a restless one. Not all my tent mates were back – it was only myself, along with Andy and Guy. The tent had become very close-knit, and it didn't seem right that we weren't all there. Since it was such a large distance to cover, the day had a 30-hour cut-off time, meaning that runners were arriving at various stages. Having been off to Doc Trotters at first light to get my blisters serviced, I spent the rest of the morning waiting for everyone else.

As it turned out, they all got back about mid-morning. It had generally been a strategic decision for all of them, except Paul, to do the long day over two days and take the opportunity of a long rest and sleep at a checkpoint. Unfortunately for Paul, he'd started the day really well, but had got very dehydrated and couldn't keep any food down. His enforced stop was necessary for his health. It was great to see them come in safely – all eight of us had made it to the final day.

My mind at rest, we were able to spend the rest of the day chilling out. As an added bonus, we all received a can of cold Coca Cola from the race organisers. This may not seem like much, but by this point it was like heaven in a can. I recall one guy dropping his, the can literally spinning around and spewing all the fluid from it. This calamity reduced the guy to tears – as if the simple can was a priceless family heirloom.

It also happened to be my mate Guy's birthday – I'd kept a card by for him for the entire race so far, as well as his present: a tube of fruit pastilles. I think he liked the surprise, even if the card was soaked in my sweat. I think it was close to disintegration point at handover.

Day five was here – the marathon stage. This didn't seem quite so daunting, considering the distance I'd covered on day four, but still, it was a lot to do, and my feet felt pretty raw. As always, the terrain was mixed, with some lovely dunes, rocks and jebels thrown in. They could have been hot coals for all I cared; I was going to get to the finish. Deciding not to break with the day four strategy, I resumed my walk/run approach early on. This was put into action across the never-ending dunes; beautiful and terrible at the same time.

Eventually, I reached the final checkpoint – just 8km to go. That was it: I knew I'd complete the MDS. I gave myself a moment to get myself together, thinking of the messages I'd been getting throughout the week, and began to well up a little. I enjoyed that remaining distance, simply running along and taking everything in. At this moment, I didn't really want the race to end.

As I approached the finish line, I massively over-thought what my celebration would be in front of the webcam. In the event, I'm not sure what I did – all I remember is getting my medal and exchanging hugs with Patrick and the UK MDS reps, Leah and Tom. I'd done it – my first ultramarathon. On the subject of celebrations, Andy was quick to remind me at the finish that I did some daft salute at the point of coming in.

Describing how I felt on completing this is hard – everything seemed so surreal. Andy and Guy had already finished by this point, and were there, waiting for me, grinning from ear to ear. It was great to see them, but by this point I just wanted to speak to Rach and the kids, so I headed to the communications tent to do just that.

'I'm so proud of you,' she said over and over again. I felt on top of the world with her words ringing through my ears, my lip wobbling and eyes watering. Must have been the unforgiving climate and sand.

After this, I waited for Paul to make it in, since, without his influence and persuasion, I wouldn't be at the MDS in the first place. Together, we toasted a dear friend of his, who he'd been running in memory of. I don't think it was the race Paul wanted it to be in terms of position and consistency. He had a few goals from the outset, and I think finishing in the top 100 was one of them. He was unlucky with the dehydration, and it's terribly hard to come back from that. I tried to assure him that he should be immensely proud of himself for dogging it out for so long while being in a bad way. I'm not sure if my words helped – regardless, he was already looking to enter again the following year.

It was done – finally, I was an ultrarunner! Only a few years earlier, I'd been coming to terms with an unwelcome bulging waistline, wondering if this was a permanent state of affairs. Now, I could say, with complete truthfulness, that I'd run across a desert.

For a lot of people, that could be – and in some cases, is – it. There aren't many further distances you can run, after all. It's probably a good thing I wasn't among their number, otherwise this would be a very short book.

Interlude 4.1

PETE AND I first met in 2011. We'd both signed up for charity places in the London Marathon and had joined some of the training runs that the charity was putting on. We hit it off and became really friendly, and our joint obsession with endurance challenges was born.

Roll on to after the London Marathon, and I was wondering about what to do next. I had this half-baked idea about entering the Marathon des Sables, as I'd met someone a few years previously who had done it. I thought I could never do it, and saw this as the best chance I might ever have to be able to do it. Needless to say, I needed a buddy for this, so who did I turn to? Pete! I remember that on the day that entries went live, I logged on to the system and paid my deposit as soon as I could. I was as keen as mustard! I phoned Pete to see if he'd done the same, and he wasn't quite as keen as me, so I harangued him into parting with his £500. There was no way I was doing this on my own.

Deposit paid, we were now enrolled in the 2013 edition of the 'Toughest Footrace on Earth': six marathons in six days, across the Sahara desert, carrying our own food, water and equipment for the whole week! We had two years to train for this.

How did he go from London Marathon runner to ultra-endurance athlete? I'm not really sure, but the journey was amazing, and one I'm honoured to have shared with Pete. His accomplishments are numerous, and I think he's quietly one of the most decorated runners in the Channel Islands, if not the UK. He has taken part in some of the most arduous and tough races out there: MDS, UTMB, Dragon's Back, Western States, the Jungle Marathon, the Arctic Ultra, not to mention pulling a car up and down the five-mile road in Jersey for the total distance of a marathon, to name but a few of the challenges completed.

What a guy, and what a pleasure it is to call him my mate!

Paul Burrows, friend and fellow
ultramarathon runner

Interlude 4.2

LIFE IS busy. When asked how I am, despite trying not to, 'busy' is normally my immediate response. Juggling work, family and the obligatory adventure consumes the majority of time available. These days, my interactions with Pete have fallen into the pattern of birthday messages interspersed with social media chats about our respective adventures. Oh, and usually an annual 'we should do it again' when we hit the anniversary of our Marathon des Sables adventure.

I climbed El Capitan, the great granite face in Yosemite last year. On more than one occasion during my training, I did question why I hadn't invited Pete to join me on this particular adventure. In hindsight, I think I could have convinced him it was a good idea. Certainly, a missed opportunity. Next time?

Pete and I met nearly 15 years ago. My first recollection of him was sat in a rather cold and decidedly uncomfortable church hall somewhere in southern England. It was the end of the first day of a multiday race, possibly across the South Downs. The race was muddy (aren't they all?), and I remember arriving at the hall feeling pretty grumpy, to say the least. After laying out my sleeping bag in a draughty corner (not a prime spot, as they'd been taken by the early finishes), I gravitated to a group who I recognised as also being on the training circuit for the upcoming Marathon des Sables. I was immediately introduced to Pete as a friend of a friend. I was struck immediately by this smiling, upbeat man, who certainly didn't look like he'd spent the last eight hours fighting through a quagmire. From then on, I had the pleasure of spending many training miles running alongside him.

Four months later, Pete and I and six others stepped off dusty coaches at the Marathon des Sables temporary base camp somewhere in the Sahara. The muddy paths over the South Downs had been training for the equivalent of seven marathons in seven days across the desert. The eight of us were to be 'tent mates' for the next week. I use the term 'tent' quite loosely, as the shelter was actually a piece of tarpaulin on branches. However, it served its purpose (kind of). My overriding memory over this time was Pete's continued buoyancy, positivity and great company. Not once do I recall anything to suggest that he was running anything more strenuous than a quick jog around his local park.

The rest is, of course, history. Pete's adventures continue to inspire awe in my household, where my six-year-old son, Jack, still intermittently questions what car exactly did my friend pull around the island, and why?

Sally Camm, friend
and fellow ultramarathon runner

Chapter 5

On your marks, get set, row!

WE WERE in the final few weeks before flying off to Spain, and the nerves were really kicking in. The days were passing by quicker than I wanted them to, and as I entered the final week, it dawned on me that I was doing certain things in my day-to-day life for the last time in months, and that there would be a fairly unpredictable experience ahead of me before I'd do them again.

Sure, I'd completed events with a risk element before, and I'd been away from home for long periods of time, but never this long, and there never had been this many risks. The situation with Rachel's health didn't help, either.

As far as we knew, the next scans were months away, and well after the date the row would be completed. Despite everything, she was incredibly supportive and sweet in the final week before I set off, and, along with Corina (Steve's wife), arranged a surprise send-off party for Steve and me to coincide with my parents' visit to Jersey. Other family members also flew in for the party, and it was a great evening in the company of family and friends and the perfect chance for us to say our farewells.

I was trying to avoid getting too deep into the inevitable questions about the forthcoming row. The project had been so all-consuming that I was just trying to switch off and enjoy some normality before things became anything but.

I can't recall who, but someone asked, 'How on earth are you going to cope with Steve for two months at sea?' It was an interesting question, and prompted me to glance over to Steve at that point, who was deep in mischief as always, while flexing his muscles in his newly acquired DragonFish vest. After this, I looked to the size of the bar. It dawned on me that the bar was around the size of our boat, and I would be living in that confined space with another person for a long time.

On 25 November, Steve and I set off, flying from Jersey to Gatwick, before jetting on to Tenerife, and then getting the ferry over to La Gomera. We decided that it would be entirely appropriate to pick up a couple of bottles of rum at duty-free for our forthcoming Atlantic row. After all, that's what sailors drink!

The second smallest of the Canary Islands, La Gomera is nestled between lively neighbours such as Tenerife, Gran Canaria and Lanzarote – its population is just under a quarter of Jersey's. I expect that it's a pretty sleepy place for the majority of the year, but that certainly wasn't the case when we rocked up there.

Ostensibly, the reason the race organisers wanted us there two weeks before race start was to complete all the mandatory inspections and make sure all the standard requirements had been fulfilled. While this was done with appropriately religious zeal and professionalism, there would still be plenty of time to kill – particularly in the evenings.

The first night was, to be blunt, a massive piss-up – there was almost an Olympic village vibe, only with alcohol in place of Powerade. Steve, never the shy and retiring type, had little problem convincing me to head straight to the Blue Marlin bar as soon as we'd checked into our respective apartments. We arrived a couple of days earlier than most of the other competitors, but Steve seemed to know a few people from when he travelled out for the race start the previous year (a 'reconnaissance' mission, he seemed to have garnered a useful amount of knowledge on the best drinking spots!). Among this number were Carsten Heron Olsen – the CEO and race director – and the rest of the Atlantic Campaigns crew.

Carsten's story was an interesting one: after his brother participated in the 2009/10 race, he fell in love with both the event and its finish line in Antigua. Clearly this wasn't a fleeting attraction, as in 2012 he took ownership of the race. After first moving the finishing line back to Antigua (the previous organiser had changed this to Barbados for the 2011 edition), he got to work, helping it to become the fixture in the rowing calendar it is today.

We ended up sitting with the group for most of the night, which turned out to be a very heavy session – the end of the night a particular blur. It was good to meet and spend time with Carsten and some of the safety team. There was some good banter, and we also took the opportunity to ask about the weather outlook and any advice on the initial route. The response was unanimous in that we should take a southerly route in the first couple of days.

At some point much later in the night as things started to blur, I glanced over to see one of the safety officers pointing a finger in a forceful manner at Steve, who was unsuccessfully trying to look innocent. 'You just wait until your safety inspection!' was said. No idea what Steve had said or done to prompt that response! I set about being extra nice to the safety officer in question.

I woke up at 2pm the next day (always the sign of a good night), and made arrangements to meet an equally groggy Steve. It turned out that he had his own adventure getting home, seemingly remembering none of it. The unfortunate outcome for him was that he somehow managed to lose his shoes, which he'd put a lot of research into before purchasing, intending to wear them on the row. They never did turn up, so the mystery of what Steve got up to that night will probably never be solved.

Having nursed our hangovers, we set about exploring the island during the next couple of days, hiring a car to do so. There were plenty of opportunities to hike, swim and explore the rainforest. It was certainly a unique and beautiful island – shades of Jersey, in some respects – and it felt like the best opportunity we'd have to do all of this; we knew everything was going to be getting slightly more serious in a couple of days' time.

The day of the first race briefing was fast approaching, and we started to notice more teams arriving. We'd all been very active across social media, so Steve and I were familiar with the faces of some teams, even though we'd never met them.

We were more acquainted with Mike Bates (rowing under the moniker of 'The Atlantic Grappler'), a Royal Marine who was raising money for the Leeds Hospital Charity. He'd ruffled some feathers when he jokingly said during a race briefing that one of his motivators to row solo was that he wanted to say he'd rowed an entire ocean, as opposed to rowing half an ocean (team of two) or a quarter of an ocean (teams of four).

Atlantic Campaigns had cleverly edited his comments, and there were resounding boos from anyone in a team larger than solo. I think some of the entrants held that against Mike, and thought the comment arrogant. However, we knew Mike, and he was simply repeating a conversation he'd had with his mates back home – it was his own genuine motivator for wanting to do it solo. Then there were The Atlantic Girls (Millie, Laura and Frankie), who we'd spent a week with back in February on the sea sports courses. It was really good to see them.

There was a real range of ages and backgrounds: City of Liverpool was a one-man team comprising Bernie Hollywood, a man whose impressive-sounding name was somehow overshadowed by his achievements. Throughout his life, he's raised over £42m for charity, and even received an OBE from the then-Prince Charles in 2013.

There was also a ladies team called Full Throttle, which consisted of Aileen, Jess, Daisy and Corrine. They'd cycled over to La Gomera from the UK, and had also planned to charter a yacht and sail back to the UK once they'd rowed to Antigua. I don't think the final part happened in the end, but they were an amazing team, ultimately coming first in their category.

Also competing was Miriam Payne (rowing under the banner of 'Seas the Day'). Having graduated with a degree in astrophysics, she was aiming to complete the row at the age of 23. Thinking back to what I was doing when I was that age, I was working in a small accounting practice and making a very half-hearted effort at trying to get through my ACCA accounting exams, all of which I was to fail due to being distracted by Euro '96. She was a remarkable individual, and was taking everything in her stride.

From now on, all the teams would be seeing each other daily.

It was a little under a fortnight from the start of the race. The boats had all arrived, with the exception of a couple of unlucky teams whose boats had been delayed, and they were all lined up in the boat park. All the rowers were ushered into the adjacent briefing tent, and Carsten kicked things off with a rousing welcome speech.

'Welcome, fleet of 2022,' he called out. 'You've all shown amazing skills and determination to get here, and now the real fun begins.' Cue lots of applause from everyone in the tent. Both he and Ian Couch, the head safety officer, then proceeded to tell us what the itinerary would be for the next couple of weeks.

In week one, we could expect a very early daily mandatory briefing. After that, we'd be free to work on our boats. We'd all be preparing our boats for inspection in the boat park, basically taking care of anything that needed to be done to include last-minute tweaks.

In week two, the plan was for us to get our boats in the water and moored at the pontoon. There, we could continue to visit our boats daily and do what we felt we needed to. The plan was also to have the opportunity to go for an open-water row to carry out final checks of all key equipment. However, these rows weren't guaranteed and would be entirely weather-dependent.

Steve and I made sure we put our name down for an early inspection. We'd had a pre-inspection with Ian over a video call when in Jersey, and felt ready to have it sooner rather than later. The only thing we really needed to do was calibrate a couple of autotillers, but that would have to wait until the second week.

That left time for one slight panic. We were routinely unpacking the boat and getting ourselves ready for the inspection the next day. As Steve turned the power on, he quickly reported, 'There's no power at all, mate.' I looked at him, puzzled, since the boat had definitely left Jersey fully charged, with everything switched off. I had triple-checked that. After further investigation, Steve called out again, 'Ah. The batteries have been disconnected. Who the hell did that?'

We found out that this would have been done prior to shipment from the UK to La Gomera, which was standard procedure, apparently. The batteries were duly reconnected, and full order was restored, although this was very slow going.

We wanted the inspection out of the way so it would be one less thing to worry about for that week. It took place on 1 December, and would involve emptying our boat entirely so that everything we'd be taking could be checked off against the mandatory equipment lists. We'd also be tested so that we knew how to use the equipment in question, and were forced to remove all of our daily food packs so they could be checked along with our emergency drinking water and ballast water. In all, there were 120 packs, each containing 5,500 calories: 3,000 calories in each pack were made up of expedition meals, with curries, spaghetti bolognese, macaroni cheese and Asian noodles being popular; the balancing 2,500 calories were a mixture of biltong, chocolate, crisps, sweets, energy bars and assorted powders.

Ours was one of the few Adkins boats in the fleet, and for this type of boat we also needed 120 litres of ballast water stored in the hull of the boat. This, in theory, would ensure that the boat self-righted in the event of a capsize. However, it also meant that our boat and all of its contents would very much be on the heavier side.

The inspection was exactly what we expected, leaving no stone unturned. Regardless, we passed, which was a huge relief.

With this out the way, we quite rightly celebrated. This involved a lovely meal, far too many bottles of red wine, and a fairly unwise trip to the Blue Marlin after that. This led to massive hangover number two, and we still had to meet at the mandatory briefing at 8am the next day.

Steve turned up quite late, and Carsten didn't look at all impressed. I recall him looking at Steve's empty seat, and his gaze then turned to me with a serious look that pretty clearly translated to 'where the fuck is he?'

Carsten had already informed the fleet that non-attendance wouldn't be tolerated, as the information imparted during the briefings was paramount to safety. On receiving Carsten's look, I simply shrugged my shoulders, and when he turned away I quickly called Steve and said, 'Where the hell are you mate? Carsten is pissed.' Fortunately, he was only a couple of minutes away at this point.

With a bit more time to kill after receiving more looks that could kill from Carsten, we sorted out the social media stuff with Barry Hayes from Shark Bait Socials, and prepared to hand over everything to him. Barry is an expert in both ocean rowing and social media, and we'd followed his coverage of previous teams. It was, without doubt, the best investment we made out of all our rowing expenses – with the exception of the boat, of course.

We also picked up all of our communications equipment from Range Global, which we'd paid to lease for the duration of the row. This consisted of two satellite phones and a BGAN (Broadband Global Area Network) device. Learning how to use both was vital, as they were to be one of our only reliable means of communication with the outside world. The BGAN was a very good piece of kit; effectively a Wi-Fi router, this would give us the ability to use WhatsApp for messages, images and very short videos. Sadly, Netflix would be out of the question.

With all the boats inspected, it was now time for them all to be transported from the boat park and lowered into the water. Again, Steve and I put our names down to be one of the first in, and that's how it turned out. It was relatively straightforward, as we were lowered in via a cradle and just needed to row a short distance to the pontoon and secure ourselves to our mooring.

In the next few days, we were able to get out for a couple of short rows. The boat felt heavy, which was something we'd need to get used to. With all our training rows back home, we never had the full weight packed, so this was new territory for both of us. Despite this, it felt very well balanced throughout, and we were happy with how we'd done it.

In the race briefing, Ian had advised all teams that the purpose of these rows was simply to run tests on equipment, and that these practice rows couldn't be guaranteed. We were mindful that we still had two autotillers to calibrate, so set about doing this. It had been a straightforward task back in Jersey when performing this operation in calm conditions, but today it was far too windy, so we had to admit defeat.

The operation basically consisted of one rower trying to rotate the boat clockwise, while the other operated the autotiller. This had to be achieved in a small time window, and the wind kept hampering our efforts. We had to admit defeat, and headed back in thoroughly deflated and cursing ourselves for not calibrating these in Jersey.

I sought the expertise of Fraser Mowlem, the race's safety officer, who told us that for our model of autotiller, calibrating wasn't entirely necessary. Our setup had steering lines attached from the rudder to the autotiller, and Fraser just advised us to think of the unit as a steering wheel, using the plus and minus buttons to steer once we'd locked on to our bearing.

The next day, we had an opportunity to head out for another practice. We were much happier with the autotillers this time, and plotted a very short route. Everything worked as it should. In fact, all of our equipment was in perfect order. After coming back in after this row, we both agreed that we didn't need any more practice rows, and at this late stage there was nothing else we could positively change on our boat, which was soon to be home for a very long time. We decided we'd use the remainder of our time on La Gomera to destress and relax. Our families would be arriving soon, so it felt great that we'd be able to focus 100 per cent on them.

In the few days leading up to the race, our families started to arrive. Rachel and the kids, and my brother Steve were all due in, as were Rachel's parents, and (rowing partner) Steve's wife, Corina, and their kids. We were looking forward to seeing some familiar faces. I was particularly eager to spend as much time as I could with Rachel, which had become even more important to me, given the news I'd received the week before.

Rachel had called me to let me know that the doctor had been in touch. It turned out that the experts that had been looking at the aneurysms weren't entirely happy with the shape of the larger of the two – after the race start, she'd be straight off to London for a procedure (injection and scan) that would ultimately determine whether she needed an operation.

This news put me into a tailspin. Firstly, I immediately wanted to be home with her to help, which, inevitably, called the race into question. However, at this very late stage, me withdrawing also meant the end of Steve's race. Rachel was incredibly calm when she told me the news, and told me that I was 100 per cent rowing. She told me the results wouldn't be available until I was more or less in Antigua, and we were basing this on the slowest-case scenario. This meant I could be with her in person if there were to be an operation.

I think she contemplated not telling me at all, but knew I'd want to know the situation. She also gave me assurance that she'd arranged for her sister, Kaye, to keep her company for the first procedure, so that put me at ease. I knew she'd be well looked after by Kaye, since the two have an extremely special relationship. The only silver lining in that godawful situation was that I knew Rachel would be in La Gomera very soon, so I could at least spend some quality time with her in the days leading up to the row.

Unfortunately, travelling from a small island like Jersey generally means that you're heavily reliant on everything being on time, since there are always connecting flights to deal with. This predictably occurred, and Rachel's arrival into La Gomera was pushed back a day, but at least it still meant we'd have a couple of evenings together.

On the plus side, my brother Steve did make it out as planned, so I was able to spend some quality time with him, making a few introductions and showing him all the boats. You can definitely spot the family resemblance with us, much to the amusement of the manager of the pizzeria next door to the Blue Marlin. However, I think he thought I was Steve's dad as opposed to his brother. In my defence, there are 15 years between us!

On 10 December, Rachel and the kids finally arrived. I'd booked all of us into a rather posh hotel on the other side of the island. I fancied a day away from everything rowing-related, and wanted to spend some quality time with Rachel and the kids, as well as my brother. It was nice and relaxing, as we lazed by the pool, had a few drinks and killed some time before dinner. I didn't want that afternoon to end, since I'd missed their company so much. I was well aware that the 11 days I'd been away from them would be dwarfed by the anticipated time of the crossing.

Dinner took an unexpected comedic twist as, on arriving at the buffet we'd booked, the host took one look at me and my brother, and pointed at a sign.

'Trousers only,' he said – we'd both arrived in shorts, with no change of clothes. Worse was to follow: our only option was the dregs of the lost property bin, the only available sizes being small and extra small. Memories of forgetting my school PE kit resurfaced. Pulling older brother rank, I took the former, and what followed was dinner with half-mast tight trousers on. I don't think I'd ever polished off my food so quickly, and after returning to my own clothes, we were able to retreat to the bar and watch England lose to France in the quarter-finals of the World Cup. Probably a slight blessing in disguise, as I wouldn't be wasting time tracking their progress!

The next day, after spending the morning at the hotel, we returned to San Sebastian and had a nice relaxing day and an early evening meal together. That night, I barely slept a wink. My mind was racing. Everything for the last two years – all the preparation and all the work we'd been doing – was leading up to this moment, just one day away. It also dawned on me once again how much I was going to miss Rachel and the kids, I'd have given anything for another couple of days like the one we'd just had together. But I didn't have that – the following day, the biggest challenge of my life, the culmination of two years of preparation, would commence.

Interlude 5

IT WAS 2020, and I'd just finished a journey that had taken me to the top of the tallest mountain in the lower 48 states. The preparation, determination, travelling and training had all brought me back to a sense of fulfilling a purpose. My time in the military had instilled in me a resolve to accomplish goals and missions – what it did not prepare me for was life after service.

Years had gone by, and I knew there was a void that needed to be filled. Having found myself alongside fellow Air Force veterans, working together to be a part of the solution for struggling veterans, the void was growing smaller. I was invited to be part of the Fight Oar Die 2022 ocean-rowing team to raise awareness and set a standard for veterans struggling with their mental health, and in some cases battling suicide. I knew that this was what I'd been needing: that new purpose. The next two years were dedicated to preparing for the Talisker Whisky Atlantic Challenge.

We arrived at the starting line in La Gomera two weeks before the start of the race. As we got to the island and found the apartment that we'd call home for the next 14 days, we set out to find a grocery store for some necessities.

We'd made it not a whole minute into our walk when we saw a tall, bald, super fit-looking guy who was proudly wearing his team colours (as were we), and we immediately knew that this guy was a rower. We introduced ourselves, and he told us he'd been on the island for a few days, and led us straight to the grocery store.

Having gotten our shopping done – which did include a 12-pack of the finest Heineken bottles I was able to find – we made our way to the checkout. The same man who helped us find this place was right in front of me, told me to put the beer on the belt, and asked if he could buy it for us. Not wanting to decline a very generous offer, I obliged. We left the store and walked back to our apartment, talking with Pete about his experiences leading up to the row ahead of us.

I didn't research any other teams before the race. It was a personal decision to not want to try to make other teams my competitors; I wanted to solely focus on my team and our performance. Regardless, when I got back to my room, I looked into this Peter guy and his team, DragonFish. I found out quickly that I'd just been in the presence of a force to be reckoned with. You never would have known from his quiet, calm and generous demeanour that this gentleman was an elite athlete. His story and list of accomplishments was absolutely an inspiration.

Ultimately, my team's row didn't go as planned, as we capsized in the middle of the night and our boat couldn't right itself, although thankfully the entire team made it home safely after being rescued by a Dutch cargo ship.

After arriving back home, multiple fellow rowers reached out and sent their best wishes to myself and my team-mates. Peter was one. Having survived a traumatic experience, only to be praised by those I've admired, has been a very humbling time in my life.

I continue to prepare for my next ocean attempt, and continue to keep in mind the character of the tallest, baldest and most generous guy I met in La Gomera. I look forward to becoming the inspiration to others that he has become to me.

Tommy Hester, Fight Oar Die, fellow competitor

Chapter 6

Fellowship of the run

WHILE THE MDS had challenged me like nothing else had before, and I got so much out of it, I didn't want this to be the last time I pushed myself in this way.

I wasn't particularly thinking about my next challenge at all during the gruelling last day of the MDS, but the day after, while enjoying the finer things in the hotel, and reflecting on the thrill of the adventure, my mind was working overtime. The Jungle Marathon, the equivalent of the MDS in the Amazon, was something I was keen to look into further. The MDS – the long day in particular – had boosted my confidence, and I felt very ready to get stuck into some challenges that I'd always believed to be out of my reach. With that in mind, I decided to set the bar high.

It was safe to say that the fire had been lit. I'd ticked off a marathon, and I'd ticked off an ultramarathon. The next thing that I really wanted to achieve was a single-stage 100-miler. I hadn't done one to date, so that was firmly on my radar.

It was around this time, in 2013, that my little journey with Steve began. As I mentioned previously, our paths had crossed, and we already got on very well. I'd been impressed by the performance of my MDS tent mate, Andy McDonald, and I quizzed him about his training regime while at the hotel in Morocco. He'd done plenty of military-based training, as well as some self-navigational events, specifically one called the OMM (Original Mountain Marathon), a two-day self-navigational event taking place in the Brecon Beacons. Steve was the only person in Jersey who was willing to do this event with me – Andy was off-limits, since he'd already entered with someone else.

A few months out from the OMM, I shared with Steve my plans for the Centurion Winter 100 event in November. He smiled. 'I fancy a bit of that too,' he said. We'd be tackling two events together towards the end of 2013.

The weather over the weekend of the OMM was apocalyptic, with a major storm coming in. We'd intended to camp the night before the event, but the field was flooded, so we ended up kipping in our ridiculously small hire car. The night was spent with the handbrake lever jammed in my back – at least I hope it was the lever. We'd both made the right kit choices for the event, which was just as well, since it was torrential rain and wind the whole way. The organisers even had to cut day two short due to the severity of the incoming storm. Rather than adding the miles back on, the day's course was rerouted to finish before the eye of the storm engulfed us. Not that we felt cheated by the shortened course – a day and a half getting soaked and battered in the Brecon Beacons was more than enough!

In this event, you just got used to being up to your knees in bog, dealing with multiple ankle twists or tripping over tussocks and other unforgiving terrain. From memory, there were no easy bits, but we worked well together and got the job done.

This event was like no other I'd done. First off, we gathered at registration, only to be told that there was to be a two-mile walk to the start line, done to the backdrop of seemingly never-ending torrential rain. A few hundred metres in, Steve slipped over and ripped his new waterproof trousers on the barbed-wire fence. To say he wasn't happy was an understatement.

When we finally got to the start, I really needed the toilet. Thankfully, there were a couple of Portaloos. Unfortunately, both very much resembled the toilet in *Trainspotting*, so that particular operation had to be carried out with great speed and care. I'd purchased from Argos what we were led to believe was a two-man tent, but once assembled we had to call this description into question.

It didn't even look like it could fit one person in. In the event, we had a cosy night, and we got to know each other a lot more than we were expecting to over the course of the weekend.

One takeaway from this time was that I realised how Steve liked the bling once he'd completed an event – he was a sucker for a shiny medal. It was unsurprising, and therefore amusing, when he was left seething after all we received for our troubles over the weekend was a cup of lukewarm soup and a hot drink voucher.

'What's this shit?' he seethed, looking at the soup, where a shiny medal should have been.

'I'll have it if you don't like the flavour, mate,' I replied. He shook his head and kept hold of it. It turned out that even a sub-par prize was better than no prize at all!

The following month, we tackled the Centurion Winter 100 together. Taking place across the Ridgeway and Thames trail paths, it essentially sees you complete four 25-mile loops, roughly moving along each point of the compass. It was a great introduction to the format, and would be my first experience of a non-stop 100-miler. Marking myself out as a complete novice, I had my MDS 20-litre backpack, while other competitors had more compact race vests. I also had a stupidly large drop bag, and did a wholly unnecessary full kit change at the end of every 25-mile loop, which just cost me lots of time. Meanwhile, Steve had his own problems.

At the 75-mile mark, Steve told a medic, 'My feet are in a really bad way, mate.' He nonchalantly replied, 'Oh, there's nothing I've seen that can't be lanced.' How wrong he was. Thirty seconds later, I heard the same medic cry out, 'Oh my god,' when Steve finally unveiled them.

At this point, I too was in serious pain, courtesy of my IT band (more commonly known as Iliotibial Band Syndrome: a fairly common runner's issue, and a rather painful one) – I'd never experienced anything like it. Despite our combined inexperience and pain, we both just about got it done within the time cut-off, but it wasn't pretty. We suffered and really had to dig in, but I think the experience was defining for the both of us, and it certainly didn't put us off.

In April 2014, I also undertook an event of my own creation: the Bunny Run. Let me rewind a bit: back in 2013 while I was training for the MDS, I tried something completely different. I'd been thinking of ways to fundraise, and came up with the idea of doing something Easter-themed. To that end, I planned to dress up as the Easter Bunny and run between as many schools and nurseries as I could, delivering eggs to the kids. I persuaded my then-employers to sponsor the event – they duly bought a load of eggs, and I plotted a route between the participating schools and nurseries to visit on the day.

For obvious reasons, carrying thousands of eggs by myself wasn't practical, so I got several volunteers – one of which was Rachel – to transport the eggs by car, while I (by now a sweating wreck, since rabbit costumes aren't exactly lightweight attire!) composed myself, waved to the kids and delivered the eggs.

This being a first-time event, there was the odd hitch. The first time I did it, the bunny-costume budget was on the low side, meaning I ended up resembling the sinister-looking rabbit in *Donnie Darko*. Cue crying from several terrified children.

I repeated the event in 2014 – this time in a more wholesome-looking costume – and again in 2015, getting much better receptions from the kids on these occasions, whose reaction was more of laughter as I delivered the eggs and bunny-hopped out of the playground.

There was still time for a funny catastrophe involving Rachel in the 2014 event. While on egg delivery duty, she somehow managed to drive her car down some steps in one of the car parks and get it wedged, necessitating a tow truck being called out to rescue it. Needless to say, the photo did the rounds on Facebook!

After that, I became drawn to more 100-milers, and started looking at other iconic races of a similar distance. This time I wanted to tackle races that involved more challenging terrain, and perhaps some climbing. Ultimately, I selected the Lakeland 100, a Lake District-based trail race, to be run in July 2014. I'd first heard about it in 2012 when I was taking part in XNRG's The Druid's Challenge. In a complete stroke of luck, I was also selected in the ballot to do the Ultra Trail du Mont Blanc, another 100-miler.

As it turned out, Mont Blanc was also in the summer – just four weeks after Lakeland. Anyone who has ever taken on a new hobby, quickly got hooked on it and decided to do their best to get involved with every aspect of it will sympathise with my approach (or maybe not, it being self-inflicted and everything). In my excitement at discovering a true passion, I'd come to learn a few valuable lessons about stretching myself – and the level of annual leave I was using up!

The thing is, you can't go into events like this 'empty'; you need to bank some warm-up events to get you acclimatised. The first of these that Steve and I embarked on was the Five Islands Ultra in May 2014. A pretty unique event – only ten of us did it that year – it sees you run around all five of the Channel Islands: the first day around Jersey; Guernsey on the second day, and then Alderney, Sark and Herm on the final stage. The combined distance of the three days is around 110 miles. Although I'd been living in Jersey for several years by this point, I still hadn't visited the surrounding islands, so it was nice to be able to do so.

As mentioned, the Five Islands Ultra was unique, and that's exactly why I wanted to do it. Due to the logistics involved in getting to all the islands over the three days by air and sea, there was a lot that could potentially derail this event, so I figured that it would be good to do it while I had the opportunity. As it turned out, weather conditions were on our side, and we were able to get to all the islands as planned and run around them.

Digby Ellis-Brecknell, the race director, organised this one very well, along with a friend and fellow runner, Lee Bennett. There were also a few familiar faces from the 'Round the Rock' Jersey ultramarathon I'd tackled the previous year, including Leanne Rive, Daniel Munns and Simon Todd. All were extremely strong and capable runners.

Running around Jersey on day one (48 miles) followed by Guernsey on day two (36 miles) was new territory for me in terms of consecutive mileage, and it was good to experience that with the year I had coming up. The social part of the race, in terms of the general banter among the ten of us, was also brilliant, and we capped it all off on the final evening in Sark with a huge piss-up.

I entered the Lakeland 100 alongside my good mate from the MDS, Andy McDonald. We identified a suitable training run for it in June 2014, which was the Peak District Ultra, a 60-mile one-day event. Taking place entirely off-road, this was aimed at getting us ready for what we might encounter on the Lakeland. This required self-navigation, so we were able to hone some of the skills we'd need the following month. The race involved a start at first light, and we were able to complete the race just before dark, so it felt like a job well done.

A few weeks later, it was time for the Lakeland. On one of the evenings between race stages, a guy called Andy Mouncey, a very accomplished ultrarunner, had been doing a talk, telling us all about his Lakeland 100 experiences. He'd achieved a second-place podium finish in two of the years he'd raced it, and was explaining his differing tactics. One of these was to start fast and then 'hang on for dear life', which is a tactic I'd grow fond of in future races. I remember thinking that this was a million miles away from where I currently was, but was nevertheless fascinated by his account of it, and I was definitely drawn to the adventure of running in places more remote.

Lakeland is a beast of an event. Not only is it just over 100 miles, but there's a lot of navigation involved, and a lot of climbing – there's just over 6,000m of ascending over the route of the course. The failure rate was high, too: between 40 and 50 per cent of entrants don't make it to the finish line.

Taking place across the Lake District, rather than going across and around all the well-known peaks and lakes, this race instead intersects some of the more locally famous areas – almost like an insiders' tour. It was like nothing I'd experienced before – even the MDS seemed straightforward by comparison. The fact that the starting pistol is fired at 5pm was very different, and the reality is that, depending on your pace, you end up going through two evenings without any sleep. For me, this was the first time I'd been tested just as much mentally as I had physically – sleep deprivation was something I hadn't had to endure since the kids were born, and at least then I could be sleep deprived while watching *Ice Truckers*, getting hypnotised by *In the Night Garden*, or some equally inane show in the middle of the night. This time, I had to tolerate sleeplessness while navigating difficult unfamiliar terrain and quite possibly climbing something very steep!

We had a challenging experience out there, to say the least. We were well rested beforehand, so getting through the first evening was no problem, and the weather was dry. Towards late afternoon on day two, we were both feeling it, and with nearly 24 hours of legwork behind us and a significant distance to go.

Andy's wife Catherine had come to meet us with a little picnic, so we spent ten minutes with her in a very hospitable location with a beer garden in full view. Ultimately, we had to crack on, and we grimaced at each other as we entered the second night.

'Come on, fella, let's get this show back on the road,' I said, as upbeat as I possibly could. I suspect it didn't sound upbeat at all, and the thought of heading into a second night was daunting. It was so grim: I had tiredness and fatigue like I'd never experienced. The checkpoints were very warm and welcoming, though, and full of encouragement from volunteers, many of whom were veterans of the event. The stark reality of entering a checkpoint was that no sooner had you reached one than you had to ultimately get your backside up again quickly and get moving to the next one.

Hallucinations were rife, as rock formations became faces of familiar people – in my case, I greeted Abraham Lincoln and Lenin – must have been my history A-level surfacing from the depths of my mind!

It was an evening of desperately trying to push one foot in front of the other, and keep some momentum going. I remember around 3am trying to traverse over a slippery ridge, and I just kept falling on my backside, stability in my legs a bygone memory. However, just at the point where all seemed bleak, the sun rose. The difference some natural daylight can make to your state of mind and will to carry on is incredible. I was well and truly dead on my feet, but the sun began to rise, and everything was lighter in terms of vision and body.

'I feel like I'm recharging swiftly, mate. How about you?' I said to Andy. From that point, we were able to pick up the pace again and just about see out the race.

Ultimately, we completed it in 39 hours, which was fairly close to the 40-hour cut-off (saying this, only 50 per cent of starters actually completed the race, so it was a decent first effort from us). We'd headed out with our MDS-style backpacks – as I had for the Winter 100 the previous year – while most other competitors seemed to prefer very streamlined race vests. I resolved to purchase an Ultimate Direction race vest for my next race, since they looked more comfortable and practical. This race was never about the completion time; more a rite of passage. We were in absolute bits after, and I'd never known tiredness like it post-event, but I'd also never known such a sense of satisfaction.

Catherine had put a tent up for us while we waited to check into our B&B. I happily passed out, half sticking out of my tent, tongue hanging out like Andy's springer spaniel Herbie, half of my face getting scorched by the sun. It was amazing to be able to complete such an iconic race. I'd never contemplated ever being able to complete something like this when I first heard of it, so it was great to achieve another milestone.

All through this, things were very busy on the home front, too. I was working in a pretty pressurised environment as chief financial officer at a precious metals firm. On top of that, Josh and Leila were both still young, so I was pretty hands-on with them. Training occurred pretty much whenever I could grab it – the odd run at lunchtime here and there, plus a long run on the Saturday if I could manage it. Rachel always blocked out Saturday morning for me to get some 'Pete' time. However, there was no structured training plan or strength and conditioning – in all honesty, I was using each event I was doing as training for the next.

I always like to be doing something that poses myself questions, and these races fit the bill. It felt like, in doing these, that I was breaking down self-imposed barriers for myself. It seemed to happen in stages – before I did the London Marathon, I never genuinely believed that I could do a marathon, so I did it. When the MDS was put to me, that was another hurdle – I'd read all about it, and instantly dismissed it as something I'd never get close to. Then I went off and did that, too.

After the MDS, my approach to picking races was a case of looking out for barriers, self-imposed or otherwise, and duly doing my best to smash them down, whether it be a 100-miler, a mountainous one, or something completely different. If a race scared me a bit or made me feel intimidated, it almost became a reason in itself to sign up and give it a go. There was also an element of making up for lost time, given that I hadn't physically challenged myself like this in my earlier years.

While I derived great satisfaction from challenging myself, I certainly didn't think I was anything special, certainly not from an athletic standpoint. My performances were bang average – firmly in the middle of the pack, and, in these early stages, sometimes further back than that. Being middling in terms of ability didn't stop me from wanting to take challenges on, and I always looked to do myself justice. Ultimately, I felt I was competing against myself, and I liked the mind games involved while dealing with the 'inner voice'.

Beyond medals and certificates of participation, what I learned from each one was that I had the mental resolve to dig in. Throughout my life, I never liked someone telling me that I couldn't do something. In each instance, I'd go out of my way to prove them wrong. The same mantra applied to the nagging voice that sometimes surfaced in each race – while I'd hear it loud and clear, there was never even the slightest prospect that I'd pay it any heed. With each challenge I completed, I felt that bit more invincible. Rather than give in, I got my head down and got it done. After that, it felt like I could do anything. With each one I ticked off, I was thinking, *What's bigger and tougher than this one?* That's where my head was.

While Lakeland was hard, it's probably fair to say that the Ultra Trail du Mont Blanc (hereafter referred to as the UTMB) is a more difficult prospect. While it's the same distance (about 105 miles), the incline is much more severe – you're climbing 10,000m, with much tougher terrain, as opposed to the 6,300 of Lakeland.

While I was still buzzing and eager for another challenge, in my haste I didn't take into account my physical state after Lakeland. This would prove to be another new experience for me: that of starting off a challenge in a state of fatigue, but not really knowing it.

Beginning in Chamonix, a resort in the French Alps near the intersection of France, Switzerland and Italy, it's an excellent holiday spot, and we took full advantage. Quite a few of the competitors arrived with their families, as I did, with Rachel and the kids coming over so we could spend a couple of days before the race in tourist mode. Chamonix was a paradise for anyone who has a passion for running or outdoor sports. There were numerous races taking place during the week we were there, and the atmosphere in the town was amazing. The best ultrarunners in the world were in town – and then there were the three amigos from Jersey.

Many months before, I'd thrown in an entry into this race, and I'd been lucky in the subsequent ballot. As it turned out, two other Jersey men, Simon Mackenzie and Shane Hugill, had also been accepted, so we trained together and stayed in the same hotel. Jersey was a difficult place to train for an event like this due to there being no mountains, so we'd often find ourselves doing ten repeats on a steep climb on the north coast of the island, which represented 100m of elevation per ascent. They were tough training sessions, but we all made the best of it, and firm friendships between the three of us were soon struck.

There must be something about these types of races, as once again the race start was at around 5pm. Given that I was faced with 10,000m of ascent, as opposed to 6,300m, this meant that two nights of racing was inevitable. I remember shuddering at the prospect of this, especially when a noisy bin truck woke me up at 5am on race day. I've never been able to have afternoon naps, so I knew at this point I'd be awake for well over two days without sleep.

On the afternoon of race day, there was an almighty downpour for a couple of hours, but it had just about eased up by the time we started. Early on, the terrain was all churned up, which made descending difficult, especially when you're in a convoy with a load of other runners with running poles clattering in every direction. Once we broke through this, we were on the move. On the first gradual ascent, at about four miles in, it was plain that I was in trouble. 'Knackered' was an understatement; I could barely move, the events of Lakeland finally catching up with me.

'I think you'll need to go on without me lads,' I practically appealed to them.

'Are you injured, mate?' responded Shane.

'No mate. I'm just shattered and need to get myself together,' I replied.

'Just look at our feet and do what we're doing,' added Simon.

To their credit, Simon and Shane stuck with me, but I was slowing them down, and I knew it. It cost us all valuable time, and I was in shock when we came to the first checkpoint and were told we were ten minutes from being timed out of the race. The churned-up terrain had been a factor, since there were loads of people behind us, but my fatigue hadn't helped the situation. I was horrified that we could have been timed out of the race at the very first checkpoint, and come all this way for very little – and it would have been all my fault.

While these events have shown me that I'll never be taking to the podium (unless I carry on running into my very old age and get a special award), it also revealed depths of mental resolve that I never thought I had. This near miss gave me the severe kick up the arse that I needed. Steaming out of the first checkpoint high on adrenaline driven by fear of failure, we set about making up time. This became a real positive cycle, since at each subsequent checkpoint we had even more of a time buffer built up. By checkpoint five, we were four hours ahead of cut-off. For the rest of the race, we stayed well above the cut-off times. Despite the gruelling nature of the physical exertions, I'd like to say the finish was never in doubt, but we could never take anything for granted. We all seemed to take it in turns to have various wobbles, but we always resolved to complete this together. If one of us was suffering, the other two would rally and bring that person back in the game.

I recall Shane pulling an absolute blinder at around mile 80 when Simon and I were in a dark place.

'I'm familiar with the route moving forwards,' he explained. 'It's a bit like a flat Roman road for the next ten miles or so – should be a piece of cake.'

This picked Simon and I up no end. In hindsight, I've never witnessed a more challenging and steep Roman road in all my life (maybe they were distracted by rampaging Gauls or Visigoths when they were building it), so it was clearly a case of positive mind games from Shane. The finish of the UTMB was probably one of my proudest moments in terms of racing.

I've never felt so knackered, and had to go to places in my head that I'd never been to before. In addition, I'd made two true friends for life, and we really had operated as a close team throughout – it was comfortably one of the hardest races I've ever done. It served as a bit of a lesson in not doing too many things so close together, particularly two massive races within four weeks of each other. Lesson well and truly learned.

The icing on the cake was that we were able to keep in touch with our loved ones throughout the race, and knew they'd be waiting for us as we ran back into Chamonix for the finish. It was the best thing to be able to hug Rachel as I neared the finish line, and absolutely magical that I was able to run over the line with Josh and Leila as Rachel followed closely behind, recording us on her iPhone. There's a great photo of me running over the finish line with Josh and Leila – you can see it in the middle of the book!

Rounding off 2014 was an idea that Rachel came up with. Despite seeing the state that I returned home in, and being a slightly disgusted onlooker at my mangled feet, she had an idea.

'I'd like to do a marathon!' I really wasn't expecting that!

This was definitely to be a one-time thing for her, and she wanted to choose the right location to make it a memorable one. She alighted on one in Greenland, known as The Polar Circle Marathon: The Coolest Marathon on Earth! A couple of our friends had done it a year before, and reported back favourably. I loved the idea of running a marathon with Rachel and sharing her experience, not to mention the idea of doing something like this in a colder climate, so I needed little convincing. My next planned race was the Spine Race in the Pennines the following year, so it was good to fit something in before that.

The race route was a 10km loop around the ice cap before a 32km run down a snow-covered track, and then road all the way back to the airport. Rachel was absolutely brilliant on the day. At this stage, Josh was seven and Leila four, and she was juggling a full-time job with motherhood while putting up with my newfound love for racing. How she fitted in training for this, particularly when both of our families live on the mainland, I'll never know, but she did herself really proud and had the right mindset in terms of getting it done and having a good time while doing so.

I really wanted to run the marathon with her, but was also excited to be in a new climate and also fancied having a go at pushing myself to my maximum. As luck would have it, I found out on arrival that they offered an extra challenge of running a half-marathon the day before the full marathon, so the day before, I duly went off and got that out of my system. The next day it was the main event, and we'd be running together.

Before the race, I just said something along the lines of 'run your own race, have fun and take it all in, and we can both go home and tell the kids all about it'.

For the first 10km, we were knee-deep in snow, and the next 10km it was shin-deep. It was only really at the '20km to go' marker that the snow levels became more normal and we were on a very gradual descent back towards the airport. Rachel was in good spirits from the off, with a big, beaming smile as she navigated around the ice cap. She was even practising yoga poses en route for the benefit of her club back home – not something I'd ever done! They had a competition to see who could get the best pose in a different location, so it's safe to say that she won that one.

There were quiet moments in the race where I knew she was suffering, which was my cue to stop for a quick picture moment and take the opportunity to encourage fuelling up. The good thing about running in a climate such as that is you simply need to keep moving quickly to keep everything warm.

As we just passed the five-hour mark, we were nearly done. Rach admitted that she was absolutely done, and would need to slow walk the last 500m. We ran past a shop, and quickly ducked inside. 'Have a moment, and take two minutes to get psyched up,' I said. 'We are finishing this race running.'

We enjoyed a nice jog, hand in hand, to the finish line. It was a brilliant way to finish off 2014, with the added bonus of doing so with my favourite human being.

Interlude 6.1

THE FIRST time I met Wrighty, I didn't realise I'd found a lifelong friend, or that he'd save my race one day. It was 2013, a golden time for long-distance running on the island of Jersey. Back then, a small but tight-knit group of us had been pushing the boundaries of endurance running. Marathons, once the pinnacle of long-distance running, were just the start. Ultras beckoned – longer, harder and grittier challenges that tested the body and mind. We supported one another as we ventured into a sport that was rapidly gaining traction and popularity worldwide. It was exciting, daunting and great fun all at the same time; and Pete was right at the heart of it.

Pete was no stranger to pushing limits. By the time we crossed paths, he'd already completed the legendary Marathon des Sables with a mutual friend of ours. I can't quite pinpoint the moment we first met; probably on a group training run on the cliff paths in Jersey. What I do remember is how easy it was to get on with Pete. He had that rare combination of drive and humility, a laid-back nature that hid an unyielding determination.

By 2014, we were lining up together for one of the biggest challenges in the ultrarunning calendar: the Ultra Trail du Mont Blanc (UTMB). With a mutual friend, the three of us set out to tackle the iconic 170-kilometre course, winding through the breathtaking and brutal terrain of the French, Italian and Swiss Alps. Pete came into the race fit but tired, still recovering from the Lakeland 100-miler just a few weeks earlier. Yet, as always, he approached UTMB with his signature calm and good humour.

That's not to say there weren't challenging moments for each of us. Somewhere on the descent to the town of Courmayeur, Pete had a bit of a hissy fit – to be honest, we were probably being annoying and winding Pete up on purpose! Anyway, he stormed past an aid station, missing his noodle soup breakfast in a rare huff. But, true to form, he rebounded quickly and was in a great mood when we caught him up a few miles down the trail. When I reached my lowest point later in the race, barely able to walk at La Fouly, it was Pete who sorted me out. He got my kit organised, forced me to eat, then kicked my arse out of the aid station and back on to the trail. Thanks to him, we all finished together and crossed the line in what remains one of the most epic finishes of my life.

That's Pete in a nutshell: the guy who gets you through, keeps you laughing over 100 miles of pain and suffering, and raises the bar every time he sets a new goal. Whether running with him or dot-watching his row across the Atlantic, Pete shows us what true determination looks like. Yet, for all his grit, what stands out most is his big heart. He has raised thousands of pounds for causes he supports – Durrell Wildlife Conservation Trust and Macmillan Cancer Support – and he's absolutely devoted to his family: his wife, Rach, and their children, Josh and Leila.

Pete Wright isn't just an ultrarunner; he's a force of nature, an adventurer, a friend for life, and proof that, with enough heart, there's no limit to what you can achieve.

Simon Mackenzie, friend and fellow ultramarathon runner

Interlude 6.2

PETE AND I first met while prepping for the Marathon des Sables in 2013. We were on a training camp in the Brecon Beacons over a brutally cold February weekend. Underprepared, Pete lent me a pair of gloves as we set off up a mountain on a long yomp with Rory Coleman. I had to finish early to get back home, and jammed the gloves under the door handle of his car. Sometime later that week, Pete thanked me for returning the gloves and I thanked him in return. It was an exchange of gestures that cemented our friendship and a signifier of the supportive relationship we've had on our adventures together.

Cue today's date, you could count on one gloved hand the times we've had a cross word in 1,000 miles of heavy-footed adventure. Pete's ability to take all in his stride and constantly 'see the funny side' is undoubtedly a gift – along with his lengthy gait, which I've often struggled to contend with at mile 80 or so.

Whether it's nature or nurture from his Jersey lifestyle, I will not know, but Pete is laid-back personified. We sat in a pre-hypothermic state on our first failed attempt at The Spine in the back of a medical truck, chuckling at the craziness of it all. I told Pete a few days later that we should give it a year off and try again in a couple of years. Nonsense, Pete said. He was already over the failure, and convinced me to return the very next year for a second attempt, which we completed.

It was here we had our only ever 'barney' – quite an achievement, having spent many hours and days in the 'pain cave' together (Pete's phrase for the dark times of an ultramarathon!). The incident happened at 2am on a frosty night, somewhere off the Pennine Way. Struggling to put the tent up with freezing fingers and a foggy head, sharp words were exchanged. I don't think we spoke for the following eight hours of yomping, but this was no novelty: we've spent many hours in silent companionship when 'in the cave' together. We laugh about the incident now over a beer together at the end of the races we still do, alongside the time we did a runner around a field during the Dartmoor 10 Tors, looking to distance ourselves from a herd of cows. It turns out we both have a mild phobia of them. Who knew!

If I had to choose one word to describe Pete, it would be 'generosity'. For example, I struggled to keep up with Pete (we've always stuck together during our races and adventures) in the Lakeland 100. It took 39 hours to complete the circuit. At the finishing line, Pete insisted I went across ahead of him. It should have been the other way around, really. Typical of the fella.

Andy McDonald, friend and fellow
ultramarathon runner

Chapter 7

All at sea

THE DAY of the race had arrived.

I left the apartment ahead of Rachel and the kids to make my way to the final mandatory briefing. The atmosphere was one of very nervous excitement, but you could tell that everyone was now ready to row away from La Gomera and start to do what they'd been talking and thinking about for the last two years.

Carsten and Ian reminded us during the final pre-race briefing of all of the sacrifices we'd made to be here, and how proud we should be at making it. Rounding things off, Carsten simply said, 'See you all in Antigua.'

Now that the moment was here, I was absolutely bricking it. After the briefing, we were able to make our way to our boats and await our allocated start time. I remember that walk very clearly, and recall Darryl from Two-Inna-Row, another pairs team, shedding a few tears. The film crew were on him straight away. I think many of us were feeling the brutal reality of rowing away from our loved ones at this point, and were very mindful that we now had limited time to say our goodbyes.

The majority of the boats in the race were of Rannoch design, and were to compete in the 'Race' class. These boats are very fast, explaining their popularity. All other entrants competed in 'Open' class, with various designs at work, all purpose-built. Ultimately, how they'd fare would depend on how the conditions suited the various hull shapes.

Steve and I both love a challenge, which, combined with our very limited budget, led us to opt for the cheapest boat we could find. This turned out to be an Adkins, designed and built by a chap in England called Justin Adkin. No spring chicken, it had four successful Atlantic crossings under its belt, the first being in 2013.

As well as all of our mandatory supplies, Steve and I had a small rucksack each containing anything personal we wanted. We both decided to row in merino underwear, its natural moisture-wicking ability helping to keep the skin dry, hopefully reducing the risk of chafing and irritation (this was literally all that Steve was wearing, the shy and retiring chap that he is), so we had three pairs each and a couple of T-shirt options, socks and trainers. We also both opted for Tilley hats, and had a couple of pairs of sunglasses each.

Thirty minutes before our race start time, I made my way to where Rachel and the kids were. I really didn't know what to say apart from, 'I love you guys. Look after each other.' I've never been one for massive speeches and, given the butterflies, I wasn't going to start now. I gave them all the biggest hugs and tightest squeezes, and made my way back down to the boat, desperately trying to hold it together. I just about managed – now it was time to ready ourselves for our start.

Carsten and Ian were at hand to untie the ropes, with Carsten's parting words being, 'See you in Antigua for a beer. I'm buying.'

And we were off! The klaxon horn sounded, and we manoeuvred ourselves out of our mooring and out of the harbour. I remember hearing my daughter Leila's sweet little voice ring out, 'Go on DragonFish!'

'It'll be a bit embarrassing if we crash into something, won't it?' I said. Fortunately, it didn't happen, and to loud cheers and applause from fellow competitors and everyone else, we rowed away from La Gomera. It was strange in many ways, since adrenaline and excitement were soon replaced by quiet and the rhythmic creak of the oars going back and forth. We made a point of chatting regularly in these early stages, but there were also long periods of near-silence and reflection. My thoughts were firmly with Rach and her next destination in London for her operation.

Teams were being set off at two-minute intervals, so for the first couple of hours we could still see other boats. We decided to row together for as long as we could so that we could make a good start, and the plan was to do this for most of the day. Once we were out of sight of the Canary Islands, there would be nothing but sea and sky ahead of us. Plenty of blue.

We'd both trained so long for this moment, and now we were actually doing it. So many people had helped and supported us along the way. Sure, there would be the communications we'd be having with the race officials, social media guys, family and more, but for all intents and purposes, we were now on our own. If an emergency were to happen, we knew it could take hours or days for us to receive assistance, particularly the further we rowed away from land. In the absence of support around us, we did what we'd told everyone we were going to do for two years, and trained so hard to do: we rowed, and gave it everything.

While the headwind was a constant menace from the off, and our trajectory dashed around a bit as we got used to the steering and using the autotillers, the first day and evening saw us tot up a solid tally of 28 nautical miles, which was a good effort on our behalf. It was a very hot first day of rowing, and we felt the exertion as we battled constant headwinds. All we had left were another 2,772.

As we sat watching the sunset in the first evening, polishing off the pizzas we'd picked up from a local restaurant in San Sebastian the day before we left, we reflected on a successful first day's rowing. The first night proved to be a memorable one under the starlit sky, seeing the occasional shooting star and watching phosphorescence in the water, as well as witnessing a huge red moon.

'Too early for rum,' Steve shouted over to me. 'Patience, my pretty,' I replied, with Steve knowing that Sunday evening was the designated rum slot. Today was Monday. By sunrise, our bottoms were already thoroughly chafed, and our hands equally sore. Welcome to ocean rowing, indeed.

Just after sunrise, Steve dug out the Jetboil, and started to heat up water to prepare a few expedition meals for the both of us. This didn't quite go to plan because of the general motion of the boat and the lack of space on deck, and it made the process of heating up water very problematic, due to the risk of burning ourselves (I, in particular, didn't have the best track record of this – my mum loves to remind me of the time I burnt myself at Scouts, Akela almost wetting himself as he told her the story of how it happened), so we ended up eating everything cold or lukewarm. This seemed the sensible course of action given that scalded hands and feet weren't going to help our rowing attempts. We told ourselves that we preferred cold food, anyway.

'The pioneers of old didn't have Jetboils,' Steve reminded me. If it was good enough for them, it would be good enough for me.

We carried on in a similar vein, rowing into headwind in extremely hot conditions. We were even able to get out for our first swim, which was welcome, given the heat. It was something we'd have had to do anyway at some point later in order to scrape off the barnacles that had become attached to the hull. These would ultimately slow our progress, so this was something we wanted to stay on top of.

There were certain conditions that needed to be adhered to as part of this row, one of which was to have your harness on at all times and be clipped on to the boat. This was for our own safety, since if we were to fall into the sea and not be secured to the boat, the consequences could be dire.

This was famously highlighted in the 2005/06 race when TV presenter Ben Fogle (rowing alongside multiple Olympic gold medal-winner James Cracknell) was swept overboard by a rogue wave, only just managing to get back on board. This was before the rule had been brought in, and highlighted its importance.

Safety protocol was key on swimming, too: we'd need to secure a line from the boat to our harnesses before jumping in. Entering the water for the first time was quite daunting. I sat on the side and pushed myself off, and it was then a case of getting a visual underwater as soon as I could to see if anything was lurking and on its way to eat me. Thankfully, all I ever saw was reassuring turquoise blue.

Then the evening came, and duly reminded us what we'd signed up for. The winds picked up, with the side of the boat getting battered by the ensuing waves. This posed two main issues: first, the possibility that it would blow us off course; and secondly, with all the missed strokes from the oars on the uneven sea, we'd find it very difficult to maintain our planned course.

We had taken four autotillers with us, and given them names: Andy, Bill, Chris and Dave, after some of our sponsors. In simple terms, an autotiller is like a steering wheel, operated via a simple rudder system. The boat can be steered manually by foot or hand but, in order to make everything as efficient and smooth as possible, all teams used autotillers. As the name suggests, this is a system that automatically controls the steering based on a bearing. However, the ocean is a very heavy and lively thing, so pushing against it puts the autotiller under significant stress, so the general idea is to swap them over regularly before they overheat.

Our autotiller of choice, a Raymarine ST2000, had been doing its job very nicely, gradually adjusting and ensuring that we maintained our planned bearing. However, the wind was strong and gusty, catching our stern cabin. When this happened, we lost our course very quickly and the autotiller could do nothing to assist us, given the force of the wind against the cabin. We were then faced with the prospect of manually bringing the boat around to our intended course and engaging the autotiller once more. The manual turning became a two-man job, and was very energy-sapping, especially given the weight of our boat. The most frustrating thing was that the wind was generally blowing the way we wanted it to, but the occasional swirling gusts were knocking us side-on.

As soon as we engaged the autotiller on to our desired bearing, a gust would catch us once more, and we'd be back to square one. It was soul-destroying, and wouldn't be the last time we experienced this. Because of this, turning our boat to the correct direction was proving impossible, forcing us to resort to deploying the drogue. This would stabilise us and create some drag, but also meant that we'd have to sit tight and wait for things to calm down.

'Well, I don't feel short-changed anymore,' I said with a slight smile. We were getting the full value for our £120,000 investment, what with all the adversity that was getting thrust our way so early on.

'Look at it this way, bud: gives our arses a chance to recover,' replied Steve.

In a way, the enforced rest was initially welcomed, and we both started to reflect on the baptism of fire we'd just experienced. On the other hand, we felt that there was a real risk of an early capsize. We couldn't help feeling uneasy.

We'd been getting pretty soaked by the constant barrage of water. This being salt water, it was particularly problematic, as our backsides were already developing sores from the constant sitting down. The addition of salt water to the mix wasn't a welcome one! We'd spent many hours training on our boat in the coastal waters off Jersey, and I'd done the same on my Concept2 rowing machine. We'd both assumed that these would nicely condition our backsides. This couldn't have been further from the truth.

Looking back now, we certainly could have thought through our rowing seats a bit more, We'd opted for basic wooden planks, and taped various layers of foam (from a cannibalised yoga mat) to them. It had worked for the previous owners, and our budget didn't allow for any upgrades here.

The main differential here was the movement in the Atlantic. The conditions in Jersey were very different, and the general motion on our backsides was back and forth. In the Atlantic, especially given the hectic conditions we started in, the motion was back and forth, side to side and continuous. This meant more friction, leaving our backsides in a very sorry state just 36 hours in.

The best remedy, despite the availability of various lotions and potions, was fresh water and air. This was easier said than done, due to the limited availability of fresh water and the difficulty in keeping ourselves dry in the chaotic conditions.

Another decision came back to haunt me. A couple of days before the row, I'd applied Veet to my hairy backside on the basis that it would make cleaning and general hygiene far easier. However, my newly bald backside wasn't coping well with all this activity, and the hairs would have been very much welcome back to offer some protection.

Then there was the sunburn – we had sun cream, and plenty of it, but it sweated out pretty quickly, so we needed to reapply to avoid burning. In this regard, we helped each other out, and would apply liberal doses of sun cream to the other's back, given that's usually the most challenging area to reach. This was actually a guilty pleasure of mine throughout the row, as Steve's calloused hands roughly massaged my back.

Back to sun cream, and I was focused on my body, big nose, big ears, bald head and the rest of my face, but also generally always had my Tilley hat on. I was also sure to apply lip salve, which we had plenty of. One area I neglected early on was my thighs, and after an afternoon's rowing with the sun beating down, my right one got very burnt indeed. It would take some time for this to calm down, and I had to ensure that it was well protected for days after, which wasn't ideal, given the circumstances!

Once conditions calmed down, the drogue was retrieved, only to find that it had been ripped to shreds. The evening's events had been frustrating, since we'd been making good early progress, which had now slowed down.

'That shitshow last night has cost us big time,' moaned Steve, but given that we were only on day two, I could only reply with, 'It's a marathon, not a sprint, mate.'

After uttering those wise old words, I reflected again on the horrifying distance of 3,000 miles and how insignificant 26.2 miles was compared to that.

After being given a leaderboard update, we saw that Minds Matter (consisting of Craig and Stu, a pair of UK-based firefighters) were leading in the open-class pairs, with us in second place. What really got to us was that if we'd managed to hold a course the previous night, we'd have clocked up a good few nautical miles, since the wind, in the most part, would have been on our backs. However, the drogue had offered stability in the chaotic conditions, and we'd at least still moved in the right direction, and not suffered a capsize. It was frustrating, but confidence was boosted thanks to the proven stability of our boat.

We were also very mindful that we were on a learning curve in terms of ocean rowing, and would be better off for every challenging experience. Little did we know that there would be quite a few of those coming up.

We were on the move again for the next few days. The wind had dropped significantly, and we managed to settle into a routine. Unfortunately for us, due to the severe state of our backsides, we had to resort to rowing one hour on and one hour off. This is generally unheard of in terms of a rowing strategy. Any longer on the rowing seat had become far too painful, so this is what we resorted to.

The obvious downside was that this didn't leave much time to sleep and refuel. Although it slightly alleviated the pain problem, it posed another one: sleep deprivation. An hour isn't a lot to begin with, but once you've factored in getting changed, preparing food and cleaning yourself, there's even less time. Sleeping was brief, to say the least. The shifts taking place between midnight and 5am were the worst, especially when wet, due to extreme tiredness, the cold (which felt more pronounced due to fatigue) and darkness. There was no getting around how horrible this was to deal with, and it was taking its toll.

The challenges in these first few days kept mounting: like many of the other competitors, we were having issues when it came to power consumption and were struggling to get our batteries above 50 per cent. We had to be very careful not to run them down too much due to the risk of them not recovering, so we weren't letting them drop below 30 per cent. This led to us cutting out any luxuries that required battery charge, and we had to be mindful when using our water maker. This led to our next major challenge, which was the reliability of it. Like everything else on our boat, we had an older model, but it had been serviced and passed all the pre-race checks. The main issue was with constant air locks, given the chaotic conditions we were rowing in. The water intake was through the hull of the boat and all the bouncing around was the cause of the air locks. No sooner had we removed one, than we would get another.

Due to the constant drain on the battery, we had to turn the water maker off and resort to manually pumping water from the ocean with our handheld water maker. This was no picnic – it took about 250 pumps just to produce a single bottle's worth. This created its own problems, with the amount of energy that had to be utilised to produce such a measly amount. We also had to do this in our one hour off rowing.

So to summarise, well under a quarter of the way through, we'd experienced:

- The risk of capsize
- Arse soreness
- Extreme sleep deprivation
- Assorted boat faults
- An enforced change to our rowing shift plans
- Now, dehydration

Both Steve and I are generally pretty laid-back people, but ultimately, the cumulative effects of everything took its toll, as we had our first (and only) argument of the entire event.

This occurred in the midst of our water maker issues, and when the pain from our hour on and off rowing was at its height. Steve was frustrated with me due to the fact that I was obviously in pain, but not doing anything about it. My stubbornness led to me not consulting the medics or even using any medical supplies. In truth, I was a bit of a liability at this point, as my mind was preoccupied with my wife and her medical challenges. I think I wanted to be anywhere but on this boat.

I sensed some frustration in Steve, and when he emerged from the cabin after his one hour off, I asked him if there were any issues between us. 'What's going on mate? Are we good? You seem a bit negative to me, so I want to see what I've done.'

The strongly worded reply was more than I had anticipated. 'You're a fucking liability, and you need to get your act together.'

I was already feeling very low, and sank my head as Steve rambled on, and I reluctantly listened. My only other choice was to jump off the side of the boat, which felt quite tempting right about now. For the time being, I was stuck in a confined space, getting told off as he delivered some strongly worded home truths.

During my telling-off, I had no issues accepting the valid criticism. Some of it was a bit cheeky, but I think he was getting a bit excitable, and Steve is never one to shy away from a good speech. I think he was trying to use it as an opportunity to motivate me. While no one enjoys criticism, for the most part I knew full well that he was correct in what he was saying, and I really respected him for that. I resolved to have a good inner word with myself and pull myself together, and we were able to move on very quickly. Before the row, we always knew we'd have to find ways to get the best out of each other, and if that required tough words, then so be it.

While all of the above sounds a bit doom and gloom, there were many reasons to be cheerful. By about day ten, despite many challenges and setbacks, we'd taken the lead in our class (open class/pairs). While I'd never really entered events with the serious intention of winning (challenging and pushing myself was enough of a race in itself), it did make us feel like we were on the right track. Every Sunday, at sunset, we'd make a point of collectively putting the oars aside and taking 15 minutes to drink rum and reflect on our successes and challenges so far. We were pleased with how we'd coped with our baptism of fire.

Sea sickness wasn't really the issue that I'd thought it would be, either – the tablets and patches did their work well. And other than the various technological faults, the boat itself was holding together nicely.

In a way, the further we rowed, the easier things would get as we learned about ocean life and became more familiar with how to control our boat in various conditions. The food we carried with us contributed greatly to our load – we were putting away around 5,000–6,000 calories a day, which we figured over time would have made a sizeable dent to the overall weight of the contents. However, we were also losing body weight rather rapidly, so I think everything balanced itself out in the long run.

There were also two magical times each day to look forward to. The morning sun always signalled the end of a hard-fought night; the feeling as it slowly warmed our faces and body after a cold and damp night, and flooded the horizon with a whole spectrum of colours, was like no other. I've always found a rising sun to be like an injection of energy for mind and body, and it was uplifting if you were on the oars during sunrise. You'd witness the ocean coming to life again, in terms of being able to see it in its full glory, and it signalled the start of a new day at sea. I always appreciated that these days, alone in the ocean, would be finite in my lifetime, and I resolved to enjoy and savour each sunrise I witnessed.

The evening sun, while signalling the start of the night, always seemed to throw out even more colour, and it was a good time to reflect on the day's events and achievements and just enjoy it.

Plus, look at where we were. We were in a completely alien environment – one we'd likely never experience again. Among the various wildlife, dolphins and turtles were spotted, reminding us that we really were far from home! We even saw a pod of whales at one point, which was utterly awe-inspiring.

Around about 22 December, the GPS went down. Annoying at the time, this would have some ramifications later on.

By 23 December – 11 days after setting off – we were able to row directly above the Cape Verde Abyssal Plain. At its deepest point, it reaches a depth of approximately 7,290m (23,920ft) – one of the deepest areas of the Atlantic. The area has been studied in great detail, providing an array of insights into the processes that have shaped Earth's crust over the years – to travel across this almighty expanse was more than a bit humbling.

Even so, we'd ended up further north than we'd planned. While most teams initially take a more southerly approach in these early stages (in theory a more direct route), we had instead taken a more south-south-westerly route, the reasons for this being our handy weather router and the fact we were finding it very difficult to actually get south with the conditions we were facing. The winds were very strong and generally heading south but, due to the messy seas with waves in all directions, we were constantly getting smashed beam-on, making progress very difficult and uncomfortable. We agreed a tactic with our weather router that it was better to make progress rather than fight the ocean, so this resulted in us staying north.

I recall a conversation we had via WhatsApp with our social media expert, Barry, when we were explaining our frustrations at not being able to get south. I explained to Barry, 'I'm an insignificant visitor here and the ocean is boss, and we've decided not to fight it. For now, we're going with it, and we're confident we'll get south soon enough.'

Our weather router was a wonderful chap called Tim Cox, who we'd met when he tutored us at our mandatory pre-race courses in Teignmouth. We formed a firm friendship, and he agreed to be our router. A weather router is an expert sat on the shore checking the weather each day and providing advice based on what they can see. However, weather isn't always the most predictable thing, and they're advising based on how they think the weather will unfold based on various forecasts available to them.

While conditions had been chaotic from the beginning, to put it mildly, we seemed to have been performing better of late, and were certainly working well together. However, we knew that some low-pressure systems were coming through, and were advised that the more northerly boats in the fleet were in for a potentially rocky ride, given how this unpredictable weather was unfolding. This was certainly going to be a very different Christmas.

Interlude 7

THE FIRST 12 days were a very steep learning curve as we adjusted to life at sea. Establishing a routine became the number-one priority, but there was a lot to learn, a lot of mistakes made and some scary situations to deal with.

The first day was a roller coaster of emotions – fear, joy, excitement, loneliness, elation, worry, relief, fear! Two years of hard work. Relentless project management. Holding down a full-time job. Being the family man as dad of three, all while spending every waking minute planning and thinking about the row. Now, it was happening. We were doing it.

And then a wave hits us like a train from the side, propels me from my rowing position and leaves me with a long graze on my back. Everything on a rowing boat is pointy and designed to hurt you.

Sleep deprivation, bum sores, homesickness and sea sickness became monumental challenges as we adjusted to life on our little boat. The plan had been to row the usually adopted routine of two hours on the oars and two hours off, all day, every day until we reached Antigua. The plan didn't work, as our backsides became so painful that we couldn't sit for longer than an hour, so started a one hour on, one hour off routine, which helped our bums, but didn't help us deal with the sleep deprivation.

The lack of sleep accumulated to breaking point ten days later when the conditions became rather sketchy and completely life-threatening if we didn't have our wits about us. Controlling the boat while surfing down a 20ft wave was new to us, but needed to be learned on the go, and quickly, to prevent us going side-on to a breaking wave and suffering a capsize.

During the first week or so, we also learned that power management was extremely important. We hadn't needed to worry about this or, naively, practise this in Jersey, as we didn't have all of our equipment switched on at the same time. In Jersey, we didn't need the water maker and the autotiller; we took our own water on training rows, and we knew where we were going. Out here, we needed the autotiller to keep us moving in the right direction, our radio in case of contact from the race team, our GPS, the AIS, navigation lights, music, etc. After two days, we saw our batteries alarmingly depleted, and needed to resort to a very strict power management plan of 'essentials only'. Music and speakers would be the first to go, followed by any cabin lights, the water maker, and whatever else we could do without while our batteries slowly restored to health.

The first weeks weren't all bad, though. We had a few wildlife encounters (whales, dolphins, turtles), experienced the wonderful feeling of dawn break on about the third or fourth day and not being able to see land. We had our first swims in the 4,000-plus-metre-deep ocean, and quickly adjusted to a naked life working on the tan lines, much to Pete's dismay. That was something he'd have to get used to.

I was the first to get in the water while Pete stayed on shark watch. I'd tied a long rope to my ankle, and had already leaned over the side to put my face in just to check that nothing was hiding under the boat. Tentatively, I lowered myself over the side while keeping a very firm grasp of grab lines mounted to the hull of the boat close to the waterline.

Swimming was a fantastic feeling. The exhilaration of the deep water, the fear, the different shades of blues, the little fish immediately in front, but then the bigger fish 10m deeper and bigger and deeper. The feeling of being able to get clean, get a bit cooler and to stretch out fully. It was a fantastic experience, but all things must come to an end, and we had a job to do.

Now, there was just the small task of trying to get back on board, which was far from easy, resembling a seal trying to climb on to a rock. Thankfully, Pete was ready to help drag my aching body over the side.

Steve Hayes

Chapter 8

Welcome to the jungle

SHORTLY AFTER completing the MDS, a good friend put a new idea in my head: the 2015 Jungle Marathon, a six-stage multiday event taking place in the Amazon rainforest. The same friend never actually entered in the end but, nevertheless, the seed was planted.

The Amazon was a place I'd held a lifelong ambition to visit, so I figured, why not combine it with running? Having read about it in *Runner's World* magazine, as well as in a very good book by Mark Hines, a previous entrant, I was left feeling absolutely terrified, but the devil on my shoulder was telling me to enter, so I did. It turns out that when it comes to doing something that I really want to do, I don't take much persuasion!

On the challenge front, the end of 2014 became a bit of a write-off when I suffered from tendonitis. This kept me out of action until March 2015, and meant that I had to withdraw from the 2015 Spine Race, which was annoying. I'd invested heavily in training weekends, navigation courses and general research. In hindsight, however, it might have been a good thing, since my adventures in 2014 had been high in quantity and low on recovery time.

In all honesty, I'd been completely overdoing it on the race front since the MDS, making it inevitable that I'd get injured at some point. At this stage in my life, all my exercise consisted of running – there was certainly no strength and conditioning, or any cross-training, so a visit to my trusted physio, Lisa Mann, started the remedy for that.

At noon on New Year's Eve 2014, Steve Hayes undertook his own charitable challenge, running 24 hours non-stop around an athletics track. He named the challenge 'Through the Years', and I was invited to join him. Given my injury, and my prior commitment to go out for the night, I joined him early on, and again from 2am while very drunk. I'm sure my support was invaluable to him and as amusing as my failed attempt to cycle around the athletics track. By 3am, I was suitably snoring in the club house.

While I was recovering on New Year's Day, I was persuaded by Steve to enter the Dragon's Back Race, which was in June 2015. This was perfect timing for me, as it would give me time to recover and get back into race mode. It would also, in theory, put me in great shape for the Jungle Marathon. Steve had also decided to enter this, so our training was nicely in sync leading up to it.

Unfortunately, life got in the way. In May 2015, I found myself out of work for the first time since leaving school. I worked for a privately owned company, and after a takeover my role became surplus to requirements. It was one of those things, but I was crushed, since it was a job I'd given many years of service to, and one that I loved. Nevertheless, I decided that Dragon's Back was still a good idea; the solution to rebuilding my self-esteem. After all, what better than a glorious multiday (and bloody tough, at that) ultra event?

How wrong I was. At the end of day one, I recorded another milestone: my first DNF. Outwardly, I blamed the recurrence of injury – a convenient excuse, and a complete pack of lies. The real issue was that my physical training hadn't been specific to the event but, more importantly, my head simply wasn't in the game. In my experience, such events are more about mental strength than physical. I recall day one being an almighty struggle physically but, nevertheless, I completed it within the time cut-offs. However, I was in a bit of a fragile state mentally and just wanted out, so I quit the next morning.

To add insult to (non) injury, I had to get a taxi from North to South Wales, costing £200, to retrieve my car. This demoralising situation was a learning experience, which I realised probably shaped me more than success would have done.

Time heals, though, and with the support of my amazing wife, we refocused on the Jungle Marathon. I say 'we', because she knows what makes me tick, and she helped me get my head straight and firmly back in the game for this event.

'There's no shame in a DNF, and you still got a 40-mile training run in,' she pointed out. 'It was the perfect training run to get you ready for the jungle.' She was quite correct – quickly leaving behind a disappointment I could do nothing about, and focusing on something I could, was the answer.

The next few months were dedicated to getting as ready as I could. The fire was burning, and with a month to go I had a good, confidence-building run with Steve at the Snowdon Ultra 50. I was now ready for the jungle and in very good condition.

For this race, I was raising money for the Durrell Wildlife Conservation Trust, who work out of Jersey Zoo. Founded by Gerald Durrell in 1959, it has under its care some of the world's most endangered species, so it was a privilege to be able to support it in some way. As part of the promotional activities for this, myself and Steve agreed to film a video talking about the race, and showing off the kind of gear we'd be wearing. Starring alongside us was a very recognisable face: Superman actor Henry Cavill. Born and bred in Jersey, he was a frequent supporter of local causes, and was an ambassador for Durrell.

Having rocked up on his moped (he happened to be visiting his parents at the time), he filmed a promotional video with us, trying on one of our rucksacks (even the Man of Steel himself thought they were a tad on the heavy side!), which he described as like having a newborn baby on your back. He wasn't far wrong.

Off air, he was a genuinely nice guy, very down to earth and genuinely interested in the race. At the end, he was kind enough to sign a Superman book I'd brought down, and address it to the kids: 'To Josh and Leila, your dad's a legend, all the best, Henry'.

While we were talking, Josh was standing behind me tugging my arm and whispering, 'Can I ask him something?'

I couldn't say no. 'Henry, do you mind if my lad asks you something?'

'Yeah sure, whatever he likes,' he said.

Josh had his moment: 'How do you get on with Bruce Wayne?'

It was a good question – *Batman v Superman* was in cinemas that year!

'Yes, we get on – we had a bit of a rocky start, but we're now very good friends!'

In October 2015, after a very long journey from Jersey – which involved six different flights – we arrived in Santarém, Brazil. From there, we took a taxi to the small town of Alter do Chão, which was where we'd be boarding the boat to the jungle.

We had plenty of time to register, drop our bags and explore the town. It was there that Steve and I met Simon Hutchings. Simon has since become a very good friend of mine, and we've taken part in a couple of events together. He'd had a DNF the year before, so was back for unfinished business. We quizzed him on what to expect come race start, and enjoyed a good few beers together, while also taking a few dips in the nearby river. I was very mindful not to urinate, since a good mate from home, Simon Mackenzie (who I'd run the UTMB with), had gleefully told me stories about a fish that could swim up there, and was very difficult to remove. I think a mallet was part of the awful-sounding solution, although I'm not sure if he was being serious or not.

At around 9pm, we boarded the boat (on a very thin, unsteady plank, carrying all our heavy luggage, representing the first chance of sustaining a major injury), and joined the hustle and bustle of finding a suitable spot to hang our hammocks. We'd be on this boat for half a day, so some sleep would be necessary.

Not particularly sensibly, we positioned ourselves right near the noisy engine, so that evening's shut-eye was not the best!

By 10am the following day, we arrived in our base camp. We were warmly greeted by the local villagers, including many school children, who sang songs and held 'Welcome' banners. We were then shown to a forest-sheltered enclosure near the village, and found a suitable location to tie our hammocks. Steve and I initially targeted a very dead-looking tree, before deciding that it would probably be a good idea to switch to a location with more lively looking trees, lest we plummet to the ground in the early hours!

The rest of the day was spent hanging out and getting to know our fellow competitors. It was easy to strike up conversation, and I found everyone very relaxed and sociable. Steve and I were camping close to Mark Innocenti, Will and Sarah, and we also got to know fellow UK competitors, Brook and Andy. All in all, there were about 40 intrepid competitors.

I've stayed in touch with Mark – now a regular on the podium in ultras, I'm in awe of how good he's become. Mark performed really well in this race also, and I 'competed' with him (if you can call trailing far behind him that!) at Wendover Woods 50 and Dragon's Back in later years.

Bedtime was at sunset, which was around 7pm. There was little point in staying up beyond this point, since you'd invariably get bitten by something. This was the first chance to sleep in our hammocks in the actual jungle, and it certainly took some getting used to. The one I'd selected was a very lightweight Hennessy hammock, and a great bit of kit. It came with sufficient netting to keep unwanted visitors at bay.

The following morning started with the first race briefing, which included a detailed presentation, safety information and practical demonstrations by the Bombeiros (army). I also had the opportunity to hold a boa constrictor, which had been captured by the Bombeiros a couple of days before. While I managed just fine, Mike (from Canada) wasn't so lucky. Having not been informed about the correct way to pick it up, he did so a tad too enthusiastically, resulting in the boa becoming suitably enraged. Fortunately, no harm came to Mike.

After a very appetising local lunch, Steve and I explored the area surrounding the village, where we had our first exposure to the dangers of this new environment. While we were enjoying cooling off in the river, one competitor was stung by a stingray. It looked bad initially, as he was carried screaming from the river with blood seeping from a wound in his foot. He was absolutely fine after treatment from both the medics and the locals, who had seen this type of injury countless times. The same guy went on to win the race, so there must have been something in these stings.

The race notes described the first day as 'a short, sharp shock to the system. This stage gives you a taste of everything the jungle can throw at you.' Shirley Thompson, the race director, mentioned at the previous night's briefing that this would be a very difficult stage, and the day did not disappoint.

As planned, I started the race with Steve. We generally run at a similar pace, so we figured that it would be good to try to do this event together. That said, we were both here to run our own races, so were relaxed about the possibility of not being together the whole time.

'When I get bored of you, I'm going to run off and do my own thing,' declared Steve.

'Feel free to jog on whenever you like, I could do with the peace and quiet,' I smiled back at Steve.

We were looking at a 5km journey to checkpoint one, which started with a steep jungle climb, followed by some very runner-friendly trails. Steve and I were soon turning our ankles inside and out every time we didn't focus, so we cut the excitable chatter and focused on keeping our ankles intact amid the vines, roots and potholes, while being assaulted by sharp branches and razor-sharp plants. At this point, it's worth mentioning the type of kit we'd opted for. Generally, tight compression tops and shorts were the order of the day, which also helped keep certain creatures from venturing where you didn't want them to. Good sunglasses, head buffs and calf guards were an equal must, as well as cycling gloves. The latter offered good protection, since you'd inadvertently be grabbing at certain hostile objects throughout the race.

Upon leaving checkpoint two, we soon encountered a particularly brutal steep climb, sweating out body weight in the severe heat and 100 per cent humidity. As we reached the summit, Steve asked me a question that halted me firmly in my tracks: 'Where are your water bottles?'

I instinctively felt for the holsters at the front of my OMM-25 pack, where I kept them stored. Empty.

'Shit.' One immediate flashback later, I realised that I'd left them at the checkpoint. What a prize tit.

My first thought was that I'd have to descend back to checkpoint two and repeat the ascent. Even on the off-chance that I'd been blessed with the ability to go without water in a scorching-hot environment, race rules state that you need 2.5 litres of capacity on you. As luck would have it, I also had my bladder in my pack, along with side soft flasks, so I had more than enough water and capacity to get to checkpoint three, the village of Takura.

All I'd need to do is switch to a different water strategy of using my bladder, as opposed to front bottles. The race organisers showed some concern upon my arrival at checkpoint three, since they'd received reports about my bottles being left behind, but I was able to assure them that I was suitably hydrated and had enough capacity to see out the day. As it turned out, my strategy of being over-prepared on the hydration front had actually paid off, but I resolved not to be so careless again.

Upon reaching checkpoint four, I was really feeling the effects of the heat and humidity. Salt-wise, the trusty S caps were going in every 30 minutes – very necessary, since I sweat a lot.

At around checkpoint four, I had a chat with Steve, and we decided to do our own thing.

'This pace is too much for me in this heat, I think I need to scale back a bit.'

'You sure mate?' replied Steve.

'Absolutely, bud. This humidity is really affecting me, and I think I need to focus on a slower finish, so I'm good for tomorrow.'

I was struggling to keep up with him, and he certainly looked like he was acclimatising far better than me. I knew I had time on my hands in terms of cut-offs, so I was playing the long game.

I found the final push of the day very difficult. I was starting to struggle, and was going far slower than I wanted. It was like hitting the 18–20-mile wall of a road marathon with no end in sight, accompanied by a tight blanket of pure heat; the perfect recipe for claustrophobia. On the plus side, my feet felt good, I had no blisters, and everything physically was in working order. Always focus on the positives.

Local children greeted me before the end of the stage, and I was able to run over the line with them, which was extremely uplifting, and a great way to finish the first day.

What was evident at this camp in particular was the amount of bullet ants. Nasty-looking things, I'd heard all about the effect of their stings – they lived up to their name. Great care was needed when walking around, and my trusty crocs were very necessary. Hopefully, the sheer ugliness of them would scare the bullet ants away, but I feared not. Bullet ants are so named since the pain of getting stung by one is like getting shot. Unfortunately, these ants don't meet their maker once they've stung you, hanging about to give you a few more. Fortunately, on this occasion, I avoided incurring their wrath.

I heard about a ritual where, upon hitting the age of 12, boys in the Brazilian Satere tribe face a terrifying test as a rite of passage into manhood. This involves a ceremony where they must put their hands inside a pair of gloves loaded with bullet ants. I much preferred the swift pint with Dad when I turned 18!

I managed to find Steve once I'd sorted myself out, and we explored camp and the local village. Back at the finish, we witnessed Will having a 'hot shot' on one of his blisters from the medics (more about them later). Steve and I were hoping for man screams and good GoPro footage, but Will turned out to be hard as nails, and didn't so much as flinch. However, another competitor on receiving the same treatment was practically levitating off the ground, his expression priceless. I also managed to get my water bottles back – I wouldn't be repeating that mistake in a hurry! I didn't want to use my bladder again, since refilling it at checkpoints was a pain in the backside, like handling an eel. There were enough slippery creatures to deal with in this environment without adding an unnecessary further complication.

During the evening's briefing, Shirley assured us that the following day would be easier, but it would start with a river crossing. I'd been looking forward to these, so went to bed eagerly anticipating this.

The first day was billed: 'Starting with a deep river crossing, and then entering the jungle for a mainly flat course.' Care would be needed, since there were plenty of plants that sting and leaves that tear, and a huge amount of snakes. While I saw none of the latter, the former made up for it in abundance.

In preparation for the river, I decided to get my pack in a strong bin liner. I had everything stored away in dry bags, so was confident that the contents would remain dry should a leak occur. I hadn't done much swim training, but figured it would be quicker to swim rather than use the rope to pull yourself across. I was hopelessly wrong – two-thirds of the way across, the energy I was expending fell woefully short of reaping the rewards in distance covered.

I switched to the rope. I was catching my breath big time once I reached the other side, as the crossing was tougher on the lungs than I thought it would be. Steve and I headed off into the jungle. However, I felt quite sick and fatigued from the moment we started to run.

'Push on ahead,' I encouraged Steve. I was really struggling to acclimatise to the heat and humidity, so needed a bit more time to get into it. With this particular event and terrain, you've got enough to concentrate on without any added pressure of playing catch-up or feeling bad about holding someone back. It was the right call, and we both knew it.

Along the long and winding road to the finish, I got chatting to a nice Belgian chap called Erik, and we spoke about how we were both easing into the event. At this point, I didn't feel like I was coping at all well with the heat and humidity, and was frustrated, since it wasn't down to a lack of fitness on my part. However, the conversation with Eric was positive, and it was really interesting to hear about his background as a part-time musician.

We also talked about our respective children and how excited we were to be able to tell them about all the wildlife we'd seen. Erik, who was also there with a Belgian film crew, had managed to get footage of an anaconda near one of the swamps we'd waded through on that day. The whole conversation, to include not having a close encounter with an anaconda, made me feel better coming into camp.

I made the finish around 12-ish. My feet were still in good shape and, once my body temperature cooled down, I felt very good physically. At sunset, I retired to my hammock, knowing from Shirley's briefing that we'd be facing the toughest of the climbs for the next day. I felt positive – the only issue was getting used to the combined heat and humidity, and I hoped I'd feel more consistent tomorrow.

The day three briefing notes stated: 'You will have some killer climbs and descents, and you will be crossing a community with the highest population of jaguars, so be vigilant. Be ready for stream crossings, relentless hills and a night-time to remember in our deep jungle campsite, where armed guards will try to keep the jaguars away. In this stage you will find the highest hills of the race.'

I liked the statement about being vigilant – I was confident enough that my small penknife and newly acquired jungle sticks would be sufficient for this purpose, while also hoping that the armed guards would try their hardest in terms of keeping things out of camp.

The stage started with a river crossing. Having not learned my lesson, I attempted it in similar style to the previous day. This time the binbag leaked, so I had the added weight of a soggy bag to contend with. Making matters worse, I couldn't seem to swim in a straight line, prompting a shout from a fellow competitor: 'Why don't you grab the bloody rope?' I obliged, and made a mental note to always use the ropes in the future, and save energy.

On the other side, I moved on to checkpoint one feeling decent enough. I duly reached checkpoint two incident-free, and left with a spring in my step. I was feeling more like me again, and I knew I was acclimatising. However, after 30 minutes of bounding along, I encountered a major problem.

Throughout the trails, there were often fallen trees – some too high to climb over, while too low to crouch under. Hands and knees were the solution, increasing the risk of bites and cuts. This particular tree required a simple step over, but I decided to step on it and jump off. I think the reason I decided on the jump was one of elation that I was finally running as well as I knew I could. On landing from the jump, my right ankle went straight into a pothole and my full body weight twisted right.

The agony was instant and extreme. Luis, my Argentine friend, was just behind me, and very concerned with what he'd seen. Our communication methods were basic, but I assured him I needed to carry on and walk it off. Inside, it was a different story. *This is bad, very bad*, I thought. I felt sick – I could feel the fattening around the ankle. Thoughts of 'DNF' flashed through my mind, but I tried to cut this out and focus on getting to the next checkpoint and keep moving, and then speak with the medics. That said, I didn't want a decision to be taken out of my hands, so would need to put a positive spin on that conversation.

In the moments after it happened, I was convinced that would be my race over. My mind raced back to day one of Dragon's Back months earlier. *I can't possibly go back to Rach and the kids with another DNF all the way from Brazil. Not after all this effort*, I thought to myself. The irony was that towards the end of my one day at Dragon's Back, I was hoping for an injury to give me the excuse of pulling out. Now, I so desperately wanted to stay in the race.

The journey to checkpoint three was depressing, since I knew this wasn't a routine twist. At that moment in time, I realised just how much this event meant to me, and how badly I wanted – and needed – to finish it. I'd come a long way to do this, and there was no way I was coming back from Brazil with a DNF. The arrival into checkpoint three couldn't come soon enough. The medics' advice (after a tiny lie from me about the pain being a bit less than it was) was to keep my trainer on, take painkillers, push on and elevate at finish. With 20km to go, I needed to get my head firmly in the game.

I left checkpoint three faking positivity, with an equally fake spring in my step, going back to limping when I was out of sight. It was the opposite of the Keyser Söze moment at the end of *The Usual Suspects*, where he leaves the police station with a limp and starts walking normally around the corner. The route to checkpoint four was one of my toughest experiences in the entire event. The heat was rising and there were gaps in the canopy, beckoning in searing heat and oppressive humidity. I remember coming across a few other competitors slumped in the shade, taking the opportunity to rest or sleep.

My ankle was very weak, and I was turning it outwards every time I lost concentration, which was becoming more and more frequent. For what seemed like an age, I continued, eventually making it to checkpoint four.

Jack, one of the medics, saw me into the checkpoint, and looked concerned. 'Sounds like a horror movie out there, fella. How are you holding up?' I think he'd heard stories of a few of us looking worse for wear!

'Toughest few hours of my life, mate,' I grimly replied, before assuring Jack that I was on top of my nutrition and hydration, and thought the best thing was to keep moving and get to camp as soon as possible. One fist-bump later, I was on my way.

There was still another 7km to go, but I was assured that there was only one beast of a climb remaining. I started singing to myself at this stage to take my mind off things – weirdly, Lionel Richie. Best put it down to jungle madness.

Eventually, I came across a stream, so carefully negotiated myself across a very slippery log (the ankle made things fun), then took a steep jungle climb and began the final push into camp. At this point, I had a rather quirky Japanese cameraman asking me questions while filming and following me. I wasn't really in the mood, and consoled myself with visions of him getting mauled by a jaguar or devoured by a giant snake.

Reaching camp was a victory in itself, given the events of 20km back. It was a huge lift to see familiar faces at camp – Steve was in his pants, oiling himself up, just for a change. This would be a familiar sight throughout the event.

It was tricky finding a spot to sleep, but Mike was fortunately at hand, and put my hammock up for me while I sorted my ankle. Sure enough, it was very swollen, so elevation and anti-inflammatory was all I could do. Cody, a competitor from the USA, offered me some super-strong Ibuprofen tablets, which I gratefully accepted. It was bloody painful, but as far as I was concerned, if it was no worse in the morning and I could put weight on the foot, I'd be good to go.

However, that was the major doubt. I'd twisted my ankle a few times playing football, and the day after was always a problem. If this was to be similar, I was well and truly out of the game. I'd never be able to hobble the route and meet the cut-offs.

The medics took a look. Once again, I told a fib about where and how much it hurt. All I needed was a short-term solution, which equated to a combination of strapping and painkillers. Ice was out of the question, since we were on higher ground (the closest source of cold water was far below us) and under armed guard, owing to the heavy jaguar presence, with no vehicular access.

Sleep came very easily, but what was great about tonight was that we were in the deep jungle, and the sounds were amazing. Once I was in my hammock, I was frequently disturbed by commotion around me as giant spiders were seen, or jaguars and even pumas sighted. It was all very exciting – so long as the excitable commotion didn't turn into terrified screaming – and certainly a different way to spend an evening!

It was one of the highlights for me, drifting in and out of sleep listening to the sounds of the deep jungle. At around 3am I needed the toilet, so I took myself to the 'hole', which seemed to be in the middle of nowhere, looking nervously over my shoulder and waiting to be eaten as routine business was performed. Let's just say that was the quickest and most decisive Brad Pitt of my life. On the plus side, apart from not getting eaten, my ankle wasn't feeling any worse, and I could put weight on it.

The briefing notes for day four simply described this day as 'The toughest marathon on the planet.' The key tactic was to get some light strapping on. Second was to find some sticks from the jungle floor from the start for added support, which were easily sourced; I was in the right place for sticks. My dogs, Flash, Bolt and Maui, would have been in heaven.

Before the start, I saw Sarah, who had withdrawn injured the previous day. Despite what surely must have been a devastating setback, she had this determined look on her face. 'I'm here to do a marathon,' she said, 'and that's what I'm going to do.'

Her ankle was in a bad way, and I had nothing but admiration for her. This inspired me to crack on, and, as it turned out, I'd spend a large part of this day with her. The previous day was particularly hot and humid, but now there seemed to be a good blanket of cloud cover. This was particularly welcoming, allowing a strong marching pace early on. The jungle floor was the usual minefield of hazards, so focus and concentration were definitely needed.

After a couple of hours, I arrived at a water station. Just after this point, I met Sarah again, and we moved along together well, chatting and approaching the long combined 2km river and swamp crossings. The 1km river stretch came first – by now, I'd given up on the bin-liner approach. The river was lovely and cooling, the only issue being the constant battering of my shins on hidden logs and twisted roots. Sometimes, you could make them out, and sometimes you couldn't. Along the river, we'd have to climb over fallen trees or swim under them.

After the river came the swamp. I noticed some people de-bagging from the dry sacks. I don't think they realised that the swamp was coming up. Getting through it took longer. It was relentless and smelly, and a lot tougher on the shins and ankles, because you couldn't see what you were about to walk on. This wasn't good for me, but the pain in my shins and knees as they received a battering took my mind off that.

Upon (eventually) exiting the swamp, we disturbed a wild pig, which fortunately seemed more scared of us than we were of it, and just glared at us from the jungle. We'd heard that these things can charge at you, and that escape is best sourced by climbing a tree. I was in no mood for this, not feeling at my most agile, so was happy to leave the pig in peace.

At one point, I came across fellow competitor Will, who looked like he needed cooling down, so I was able to baptise him at the side of the road with some spare water. He had a good tactic of covering distance early on before the heat rose, after which he'd slow down and manage his body temperature accordingly. From this point, it was a case of following a dusty track with a few modest climbs. I saw the day out with Sarah, and we were both very happy to make it to the finish at around 4pm.

We'd be staying on a beach, so I found a suitably scenic place to hang my hammock, and then had a much-needed wash. I hadn't done this the previous day, so this was extremely welcoming. Steve was already in the water. Never one to whisper, he bellowed out, 'There he is – Pasty Pete and his jungle tan. Come and join us!' I duly waded in to be entertained by the semi-naked Welshman, regrettably not for the last time in my life.

After the day before, when I finished close to darkness, it was nice to have the time to catch up with everyone in daylight and have a good wash. It was funny to see Takashi Okada, a professional Japanese wrestler, come in. He was carrying a massive backpack (must have been over 20kg). He was very popular with the Bombeiros, and shortly after getting in, he had his Spider-Man mask on, striking a pose and getting involved in photos with them all. Andrew (one of the medics) had heavily strapped my ankle, replacing the light strapping I had before. It now felt very supported.

As per the briefing notes, the fifth day was simply described as: 'The long one.' It lived up to the moniker.

It started with the mandatory force-feeding of porridge. I made the mistake of having porridge every day at the MDS in 2013, and I'd done it again. At least I'd left the macadamia nuts behind this time.

We were off at 4.30am. The first section through checkpoints one and two was straightforward, the terrain mostly dust track. I saw plenty of creatures – you could see the eyes of spiders, and there were snakes everywhere. Since I felt good, and it was cooler by jungle standards, I wasn't taking too long at the early checkpoints, and pretty much sailed through both of those.

After passing through a very picturesque beach, I entered the jungle, where I started to follow the yellow tape that was hung from trees to show us the route. This was proving hard, since following pale yellow tape in a jungle of many shades of green can be tricky. Also, the marking seemed slightly more casual than previous days, and I kept missing turnings and having to backtrack to pick up the trail. In fairness, I have form for getting lost in really obvious situations, so I can't blame the race organisers.

All of a sudden, I noticed an almighty smell of cat's piss, and a long, clear growling sound close to my left-hand side. I looked behind slightly nervously, and Luis, who was just behind me, said, 'Jaguar,' and indicated that we should move on swiftly. That sounded like a pretty good idea – I duly obliged, although not before taking a selfie (I looked pretty frightened). About half an hour later, the same thing happened, this time on my right-hand side. I thought that was odd, and was also getting a bit concerned about inadvertently angering the local jaguar population.

After another 30 minutes, that double growling episode started to make sense when we bumped into Henrique and Marlon walking towards us. After much debate, Luis and I realised that we must have somehow turned back on ourselves during one of our many corrections on missing tape markings. I was gutted, figuring that this was probably going to cost me at least two hours, pretty much ruining any chance of making the cut-off. That would be my race over.

We stuck with Marlon and Henrique, and upon eventually leaving the jungle, Luis and I turned left on to a road for the final 10km to checkpoint four. However, I'd been stuck in the jungle getting lost for far too long, and the heat had taken its toll. I saw Will sitting at the side of the road in the shade, and decided to join him. I wasn't feeling good at all. Luis pushed on, and I wished him well. Will told me there was a truck moving up and down the road delivering water, but unfortunately it never showed up. I needed water big time.

Temperatures were up to 45°C, and my body temperature was rising. I was sticking with Will, who was encouraging me to stop regularly. I was elevating my feet and lifting my top up, basically trying anything to release body heat. It was ridiculous, and I was having to stop every 15 minutes. Eventually, after another enforced stop, I tried to get up. I saw black spots, and felt very dizzy. Will took one look at me, and his face fell.

'Sit down, now,' he said. I obliged. He could hear some music not far down the road, and went to investigate, seeking water to cool me down.

Shortly after, he returned, and I was relieved to hear that he'd found a stream further up. This, bizarrely, was near checkpoint four, but the race route dictated that we had to make a right-hand turn and a 5km loop before we could check into checkpoint four. Regardless, we decided to cool off before the loop. Will pretty much ordered me to get in the stream. I duly stripped off, and remained there for a good hour shivering away, allowing my body to cool those vital degrees.

Before entering the stream, I was basically talking bollocks, constantly commenting on the amount of weird fish in the stream. Will kept telling me there were no fish. As well as hallucinating about colourful fish, I was in strong denial of just how bad things had got for me. Will was an absolute legend, and made sure I stayed put for long enough to get my body temperature down and rehydrate. After this, we pushed on together and completed the 5km loop to checkpoint four. By this time, I could talk sensibly again – I kind of sensed that Will was keeping a careful eye on me in that respect!

After this, Will and I pushed on in the dark for the final 9km to checkpoint five. Along this route there were plenty of spiders and snakes to step over. We made it to camp at around 9pm. At 60km, the day had tested me to my limits and put me in a situation I'd never been in before. However, I'd made it, and, psychologically, tomorrow was only 50km, so this was a massive positive. Surely it couldn't be as bad as today.

Sleep came extremely easily, which wasn't surprising, given that I'd been well and truly pushed beyond any limit I'd ever encountered. I'd packed my bag the previous night, so I got up at 5.30am in anticipation of a 6.30 start. There were no briefing notes for day six – we had two days to get the long day done and, on account of the shenanigans the day before, I needed this second day.

Since the previous day had taken me so long, any thoughts of a highly placed finish had firmly left my head – it was all about getting this 50km done and hopefully making it to camp as soon as possible. The final stage was to be a 24km flat course along a beach, so the 'easiest' stage of all. That said, there was a massive task ahead, and I was taking nothing for granted, based on the worsening state of the ankle and the previous day's issues with the heat.

I started the stage with Luis, Joel and Steve, and tried to match their pace through the jungle trail. Again, it seemed very hot, so my initial focus was to get some good mileage cleared early on. The jungle trail was the usual affair of hostile terrain and some vicious climbs and ascents – just when you needed them least.

After some time, we reached what looked like a huge river crossing, but this time there was no rope. A boat was midway across, and the guys on board were waving their arms. The crossing was huge and deep – there was no way I was swimming across with no rope. We then remembered that this was the part where a boat was supposed to take us across. That was the boat, but in true comedy fashion it had broken down. Fortunately, the small media boat offered to take us across the river to checkpoint eight.

I was with fellow competitor Christoph now, and pushed on to checkpoint nine. There was now only 20km to go – the end of this stage was in sight. The march on to checkpoints nine and ten was comfortable and mostly flat. It had its challenges, like when we had to clamber across quite a few boulders along the beach. However, after the monotony of the flat beach, it was fun to do some climbing. En route to checkpoint ten, it was clear that we were going to make that at sunset, but would probably have to do checkpoint ten to the finish in darkness.

Jack, another medic, said at checkpoint ten that the distance was 4km to the finish – a case of following the coast. Sounded simple enough! We left, but everything became very tricky in the dark. It was hard to follow the tape, and there was nothing highlighting the route. During this stage, a huge blister that had formed on my right sole burst, leaving me in absolute agony. I needed Christoph's poles to move forward for a short while.

After two hours of this nonsense – remember, it was only 4km – we were lost. Christoph and I were bickering a little by this point, with different theories on which direction we should head in. The only thing we really agreed on was that we should stick together. Eventually, we were able to pick up the trail, and knew we were on our way to the end of this stage. I remember arriving at the finish feeling absolutely fucked, to put it bluntly. The previous 48 hours had been very hard physically and mentally, but I'd made it. I was so proud of myself.

Geoff and Sue were absolute legends, and sorted out my hammock for me while I had my feet seen to by Amy. I'd done this for Geoff at the end of a previous stage after he came in looking in a bad way, and I was really touched when they repaid the favour. The poor girl in the medic team had the unfortunate task of washing my feet and smelling my toxic odour. There was also no way my calf guard could be taken down over my ankle due to the size, so it was cut off and disposed of.

I was absolutely buzzing, though. There was no way I was ready for sleep, and I spent a few hours seeing in other competitors and just reflecting on everything. There was an element of sadness, since I knew this was the last night in the jungle camp, and I was getting very used to this way of life. I stayed up with Sarah until just after midnight, hoping to see Carl come over the line, but admitted defeat at 12.30 and retired to my hammock. I didn't see anything of Steve – I think he'd somehow sourced a bottle of whisky and was busy suckling on that in his hammock.

I was up and about quite early, still wired from the previous day, so decided to get my feet sorted by the medic, Amy, early on. I found Steve, and we sat for 30 minutes exchanging harrowing tales of the previous 48 hours. Steve, Simon and Mark had all had their own fun and games, getting lost numerous times due to a lack of course markings, climbing over massive boulders, having to cross a piranha-infested stretch of water, and adopting two stray dogs en route.

We found out that the race start was pushed back to around 10am, so there was plenty of time to get ready for the final push. Viewing the day as a bit of a fun run, I decided to run as much as I could, since prolonged injury post-race didn't really matter to me. By now, the pack was as light as it was going to get and, after taking a teary farewell picture of my crocs (the wife would be pleased), I was ready to get started. It was a great atmosphere at the start, and after the usual countdown, we began.

I got off to a hobble-like start, but before long was in a good running routine. Today was all beach – it was flat, and we had a few water crossings thrown in. I spent most of the run doing my own thing and thinking over the whole event. I had numerous conversations along the way with fellow competitors I was either passing or being overtaken by. Pretty much everyone I spoke with was dreaming of an ice-cold beer at the finish, along with some pizza.

Given that we were on the beach, we were very exposed to the heat, which again seemed to be in the 40s. That part was tough going, but today was the final finish, and a cool beer awaited me. The finish into Santarém came sooner than I thought, and after clambering over a beach wall I suddenly saw the finish line. After a very unexpected wobbly-lip moment, I composed myself and ran for the finishing line.

It was truly amazing to cross the line, and Shirley was on hand to place my clay medal around my neck. Sue and Geoff were there also, and to my right was a packed bar with some very ecstatic competitors who had finished before me. Steve was quickly on the scene after I'd given Shirley a big hug.

'Give me that pack, young man,' he said as he smiled, and then gave me the biggest man hug. He followed it up with, 'Your round bud. We're all getting thirsty up there.'

It was certainly the time to have a beer with the rest of the jungle family, with whom I'd shared the most amazing, tough and uplifting experience.

Midway through the first beer of many, I broke off to call Rachel back home. Cue wobbly voice and watery eyes as I told her I'd only gone and completed it.

'We've been tracking you all the way, and are so proud. We love you.' Those words really set me off, and composure was needed before returning to beer.

Slightly different in tone was the reply from my father when I was telling him how it all went. Already a bit nervous for my welfare in the Amazon, my regaling of having to lay down in the river brought out the concerned father in him: 'For Christ's sake Pete, you're a father, you have a family to think of!'

So there it was – another challenge ticked off. I'd travelled across a desert, and now I could add the rainforest to the tally of extreme environments I'd experienced.

Where the MDS had been a rite of passage, the jungle had been far tougher. The environment was wholly unforgiving, and there was an awful lot that could potentially happen between stages. It's safe to say this event didn't have a huge safety wrapper, but I knew all of that before signing up and went in eyes wide open.

The event mentally challenged me like no other in terms of dealing with injury – there's a picture of my foot in the days after this event in the middle of this book. I well and truly exorcised the demons from Dragon's Back, and immediately started thinking about the next challenge. This was already entered: Cape Wrath, the sister event of Dragon's Back. Game face on.

Interlude 8.1

PETE – one of the most humble, unassuming, resilient and nicest blokes I've ever met – also completes some of the most gruelling and toughest challenges out there. And he does so with a smile!

I first met him in 2015 during the Jungle Marathon. I was new to the ultra world, having only completed the Oner, a 78-mile event along the Jurassic coast. As I found out later, Pete had completed this one also, but five hours quicker than I had.

I never got to run with Pete during the Jungle Marathon, as he got injured very early on. For sure, many people would have dropped out. This race had almost everything: water crossings, mud, intense heat, humidity, swampy bogs, animals and frickin' nasty plants. Pete made sure he finished the event, and this determination was one of the things that stuck with me: his ability to plough on through when faced with these challenges. His mind had the ability to overrule his body. I took that going forward.

We kept in touch, and competed in a number more events together over the years. One of these was the Vegan 3000 – an event that encompassed the highest 15 peaks in Wales. The first part of this event involved heading straight up to the summit of Snowdon and then crossing Crib Goch.

Now, my relationship with heights is not good, to say the least. When I started crossing, the fog and cloud came in, leaving me only able to see my hands gripping the top of the rock face. I froze, unable to see below my waist, the way forward or back, and I started to panic a little. Then, as if by magic, I heard Pete's voice. He and Brook, another mate from the jungle, stayed with me until we crossed Crib Goch. My Facebook picture is that moment, crossing with Pete shepherding me from behind. He didn't have to do that; he could have kept going. That race was another that Pete finished, even though he was not, by his own admission, in great shape. Another event where his mindset wouldn't let him quit.

During my conversations with Pete while racing, every now and then you'd discover that he'd finished this race and that race – races that I had on my list to do. You could not wish for a better person to chat to.

With each event I did with Pete, I was amazed by how many people he knew. He seemed to get on with everyone, whether he ran with them for a few hours or a few days, it didn't matter. It's hard not to be a little bit in awe of Pete and his achievements – they're impressive, to say the least.

Throughout all Pete has done, there's a humility, he never brags, and he's one of the nicest blokes you could meet. He is 100 per cent the person you want to end up running with during a race – he'll get you through. I look forward to our next race together.

Simon Hutchings, friend and fellow
ultramarathon runner

Interlude 8.2

I FIRST met Pete at the Jungle Marathon. I was completely out of my depth, with it being one of my first ultramarathons, and Pete and his good friend Steve made up part of the small UK contingent. I immediately warmed to them both, what with their cheerful characters and far superior experience in such events.

As the week progressed, the camaraderie was fantastic, as it tends to be when you all face a challenge together, and we all got to know each other very well. I remember Pete being extremely calm and unwavering at all times, with a natural quiet confidence and determination that certainly rubbed off on the rest of us, and no doubt will have benefited him in all his incredible challenges since. He's clearly a strong family man, reliable, with a big heart and a real can-do attitude.

In the years since, we've crossed paths many times through running and crewing (Dragon's Back, Thames Path 100 and the Wendover Woods 50 spring to mind), and he always had a keen interest in how my race was going, despite the immediate challenges we sometimes can all face in an ultramarathon.

I've followed Pete's continuous epic challenges with a keen interest over the years, and what a diverse mix of challenges he has put himself through! I recall him pulling a car, an epic Atlantic row with his buddy Steve, and most recently in 2024, a 100-mile 'grand slam' running all four of Centurion Running's 100-mile races in the same year. There's nothing this man cannot put his mind to.

The row in particular caught my attention, not least because it sits right at the top of all of his challenges. The thought of him and Steve, day after day on the open ocean, battling with sleep deprivation, strong sea currents, weather, and with certain vital pieces of equipment malfunctioning, would have tested their mental fortitude to its limit. There's no doubt that they'd have had to draw on every strand of their brotherly bond to keep going. It was truly awe-inspiring.

It's also worth noting that both Pete and Steve have raised a huge amount of money over the years for great causes close to their hearts and it appears that they, very deservedly, have become minor celebrities back in Jersey for all their endeavours.

If one thing is for sure, Pete isn't one for sitting down for very long, and I look forward to following his next epic adventure through 2025 and beyond.

Mark Innocenti, friend and fellow
ultramarathon runner

Chapter 9

Christmas in the cabin

WITH THE festive season heading towards its big centrepiece, Steve and I were feeling pretty optimistic.

This was reflected in the daily mileage we were putting in. Between 17 and 23 December, we were averaging just over 60 nautical miles a day – a decent innings that we were pretty happy with and that helped make us the lead boat in the open-class pairs category. It's safe to say that Steve and I were in good spirits, and our first-place position was helping with this. It was almost enough to make us forget the excruciating pain in our backsides.

Even so, we weren't quite on the course that we wanted – at this point, we were the most northerly boat in the fleet. This prompted a phone call from the head safety officer, Ian Couch.

'Hi, I just wanted to ask why you guys are so far north?'

'The fishing was better,' replied Steve.

As I touched on earlier, we'd been attempting to 'go' with the conditions rather than fight directly against them, which saw us heading in a more south-south-westerly direction.

The lack of available GPS didn't help, either. Apart from Tim, our weather router, along with our trusty manual compass, we were effectively flying blind. Taking the guide of a compass bearing was better than nothing, but the wind's direction and strength was affecting our direction of travel. Without GPS, we really didn't know the exact line we were following. It was frustrating for us, and frustrating for Tim.

Christmas Eve gave us a bit of time to chill out. We recorded some video messages and chilled out on the deck together with some rum. Considering how up and down the previous few days had been, it was nice to be able to sit back and reflect on things, with 'Do They Know It's Christmas?' blaring over the speakers.

We both enjoyed a good swim and took the opportunity to stretch our limbs. Accommodation on an ocean-rowing boat doesn't really allow you the luxury of stretching out, so being in the open water is the only chance you get to do this. Whenever we enjoyed our rum on deck, we tried to reflect on something positive, while at the same time addressing challenges we may have encountered and discussing what we'd learned. In this instance, we were enjoying being in the lead and were equally happy with our progress over the previous week.

This optimism prompted me to declare to Steve, 'I think we'll have this race wrapped up in around 45 days, mate.' Steve was equally optimistic, and we felt that all the challenges we'd encountered so far, along with subsequent learnings, would certainly put us in good stead for the remainder of the row.

Me and my big mouth. Christmas Day would bring us the very opposite of Christmas cheer.

The problems started early on in the morning when, during one of the day's first shifts, I heard a splash, shortly followed by some swearing. Looking outside, it turned out that Steve had managed to drop the portable solar panel over the side, which he was in the process of chastising himself for.

'You alright mate?' I asked as positively as I could, knowing full well that he wasn't, given the look on his face.

'I've lost the solar panel,' he grimly replied.

'Don't beat yourself up, bud. It's not like we don't have other options to charge things,' I replied, pointing to our solar panels on the stern and bow side. Ironically, we'd only learned how to use the portable panel the day before, and it would have come in quite handy with the charging problems we were yet to face at this point. However, these things happen, and it wasn't to be the last item we'd lose to the ocean depths.

Even so, we managed to make a day of it in between the rowing, taking the time to open some presents from friends and family. We treated ourselves to some chocolates, plus some Havana rum and Malibu that Frankie, Mille and Laura (from trio team 'The Atlantic Girls') had given us. Rachel had given me some red wine and cheese, which I decided to save for my evening shift. Each of the chocolates had a piece of paper containing a joke wrapped around them, which provided a good lift. It was standard Christmas cracker fare, but in our tired, sleep-deprived state, they seemed a lot funnier.

At this point, closing in on 2,000 miles to go, we were full of hope that we'd be able to angle our direction further south in line with where the rest of our competitors were heading. While conditions were slightly more tricky than in the previous week (early on in the day, it was like rowing through treacle at times), we still averaged about 50 miles. However, today the sea was looking and feeling very confused, with waves moving in all directions, and gusts starting to pick up.

I'd kept my watch on UK time throughout the row, and around mid-afternoon, while in the stern cabin, I made a call to Rachel and my other family members via the satellite phone. I assured Rachel that I was okay and sought the assurance that everyone else was fine, including our three dogs. I missed them all more than ever, but kept my emotions in check on account of not wanting to put too much on them. I sensed that their Christmas was far more subdued than it usually would be, on account of the nerves from checking regular updates on the tracker.

Next on the list was my parents. The reception seemed pretty decent, and I'd coincided my call with their Christmas dinner. The phone was duly passed around the table, as I heard laughter and the chinking of glasses in the background. Envy was certainly an understatement, given that my own dinner had comprised lukewarm macaroni cheese. That said, I finished the calls feeling quite upbeat and knowing they were all very proud of our progress to date.

This all changed when I heard a knock at the cabin door, which usually indicated that Steve wanted to give me an update on something, so I duly opened the hatch.

The look on Steve's face that greeted me was that of someone who had aged 20 years in about an hour.

'You'd better get out here, mate. The conditions have gone crazy, and it's going to need both of us to deal with it.'

Shit. Out I went. It turns out he wasn't exaggerating as, shortly after, things started to get a bit scary. The wind speed had picked up significantly, prompting the very necessary consumption of a few shots of rum to fortify our nerves.

By late afternoon, it had reached speeds of around 30 knots. The wind, waves and swell were now coming at us beam-on, and we were getting well and truly battered and bruised. The winds were very strong and heading south, but everything was very messy and confused, making any semblance of controlled progress impossible. Strong gusts would catch our stern cabin and put us side-on to the waves, leaving us at real risk of capsizing.

Our upbeat Christmas music had been replaced with the sound of howling wind, and we were getting absolutely soaked as waves lashed over the deck. It was a stark reminder of how quickly everything can change, and how you could take nothing for granted. I remember thinking what a good day it had been so far, and the subsequent swift change in our circumstances. I was quickly learning about the unpredictability of ocean life as the Christmas cheer from 15 minutes earlier swiftly evaporated, to be replaced by the absolute terror of the rapidly changing and rather threatening sea state. However, fear does tend to keep you very focused – which was just as well, as we certainly needed to be.

With conditions continuing to worsen, we both agreed that it was time to deploy the drogue for the second time in the race, and retreated to the cabin. At the time, it didn't feel like this was such a bad thing – it was Christmas, and we'd just spent the past couple of hours getting completely battered by the elements. It felt nice to get some sanctuary and recharge via some enforced R&R.

Little did we realise that it would be another four and a half days before we'd be able to row properly again, during which time we'd be mostly confined to the stern cabin.

The cabin wasn't quite the safe haven that we imagined it would be – it was absolutely terrifying, to say the least. At times, it felt like a sledgehammer was battering away at the side of the boat. Coupled with some very violent sways, we were convinced that it would be a matter of time before the inevitable capsize. From what we've since heard, this happened to at least three teams during this particular storm.

We adopted a top-to-toe strategy in terms of cohabiting the cabin.

'Not exactly the time to start watching *Titanic* is it, mate?' I said to Steve. For some reason, we'd downloaded that as part of our on-boat film library.

While we didn't share the capsized teams' fate, there were some casualties. In our haste to retreat to the cabin, many of our Christmas gifts were left on the deck. When I ventured back out to retrieve my red wine, cheese and Twinkie bars (either a winning combination, or they all just taste better together when you're in the middle of the ocean), I discovered that they'd all been swept overboard. The sea is a cruel mistress indeed.

Being stuck in the cabin was, to put it bluntly, pure misery. It was like living in an airing cupboard – there was no space, with the both of us lying there, and very little in the way of comfort. In fact, we were both developing mattress sores from lying down for so long.

All of this was set to the soundtrack of Steve playing his harmonica, which had been a Christmas gift from his kids. Unfortunately for me, Steve had retrieved this from the deck, so it hadn't shared the same fate as some of our other Christmas gifts.

While Steve and I are good friends, being stuck together with nothing to occupy us for days on end was enough to challenge anyone's endurance for one another. We both had to continually adjust ourselves, since no position was comfortable, and had to source makeshift pillows, since our inflatable ones had either burst or been swept overboard.

The substitutes included sponges, shoes and each other's body parts. There wasn't a whole lot of conversation happening during this enforced stay, aside from mutual wishing that we wouldn't capsize, and praying to get rowing again soon.

At one point during Boxing Day, as we both woke from a slumber, we tried to move, only to discover that our backsides were effectively glued together by sweat. The subsequent unpeeling still makes me shudder to this day.

To make matters even worse, we were out of distractions. While still on land, I'd made a point of downloading a few good viewing options on to my brand-new iPad, should we end up in the kind of predicament we found ourselves in now. There was all sorts on there, including *Titanic*, as I mentioned earlier. While this may seem a questionable choice, considering the subject after, my logic was sound: if we watched it at a low point, we could count ourselves lucky that we weren't in Leo's predicament. It's always a good tactic in endurance racing: pick out someone that's in a worse position to make yourself feel slightly better.

In this situation, however, I decided that *The Inbetweeners* would be just the tonic. I reached out for my iPad. 'Here's a little something to pass some time and lift spirits,' I said to Steve.

I pressed the power button, only to find that the bloody thing wouldn't turn on. It had been fully charged on leaving La Gomera, and hadn't been used yet. On closer examination, the charging port was showing signs of corrosion. I'd never get to use that brand-new iPad. Only just out of the box, and it was already knackered. Another victim of the ocean.

As the days ticked by in that sweat-soaked cabin, we came to realise that a whole bunch of our equipment had met the same fate – Kindles, iPods, chargers. All went kaput. We did have everything in protective bags, but that didn't seem to matter. The cabin was absolutely soaked, and horrendously grotty.

For each of the four days, we dearly hoped that it would be our last in the cabin. We'd venture out on to the deck, try to get going, get knocked side-on to the wind as gusts caught the stern cabin, and then quickly have to abort. The physical exertion in trying to turn the boat so we could catch the southerly wind was huge, and our shoulders and arms were burning. We were sure that our tendons were going to get ripped at some point. Soul-destroying didn't quite cut it. We just couldn't get anywhere, and every day was starting to feel like Groundhog Day.

We were both pretty low, and were trying to make the situation as light as we could by chatting about it openly and honestly. At one point, Steve came in after a soaking and declared, 'Mate, I really thought about hanging myself today.'

I probed him a little on how that would actually work on an ocean-rowing boat. He explained that he'd do it off the side of the boat so his demise would be a combination of hanging and drowning. I explained that it probably wouldn't be the quickest of deaths – maybe getting eaten by a shark might be a more sensible option? He replied that he wanted to give me an opportunity to enter him for the Darwin Awards so that he could be remembered for all time. That did make me chuckle. Always the attention seeker.

Despite the previous few days being less than fun on several occasions, something often pops up to remind you that somewhere, someone else is worse off.

On 29 December, we received distressing news: Fight Oar Die, a four-man team from the USA, had been forced to drop out of the race. I'd stayed next door to them in my apartment for a fortnight in La Gomera, and had a lot of time for them. They'd already been dealt a cruel hand back on land when their boat's arrival on the island was delayed, costing them days of preparation time. Yet, worse was to come: during the storm, their boat capsized, but for whatever reason it didn't self-right, forcing them to deploy the life raft from their capsized boat. They did everything they'd been trained to do, and were heroes for doing so. With the help of the coastguard-liaising Atlantic Campaigns, the crew were eventually rescued by a Dutch bulk carrier that was bound for Canada. This news just highlighted the danger we knew we were facing at this time.

'Jesus! Those guys just haven't had any luck, have they mate? It puts our own position into perspective,' I said to Steve.

He pointed out, 'They've actually been lucky. Do you know what the actual chances of getting picked up by a rerouted vessel is, particularly given their location?'

Steve was indeed correct. While Fight Oar Die had indeed put their training into practice, the odds of survival would have been firmly stacked against them.

All in, we averaged around 25 miles per day over those four days. It was absolutely gut-wrenching to see the progress we'd fought so hard to make being upended, and knowing that there was nothing we could have done about it. The only real crumb of comfort was that, again, despite some close calls, the boat hadn't capsized, and we were still edging closer to Antigua.

Who knows what was in store up ahead? Was the worst over? Whatever was to come, there was only one way forwards.

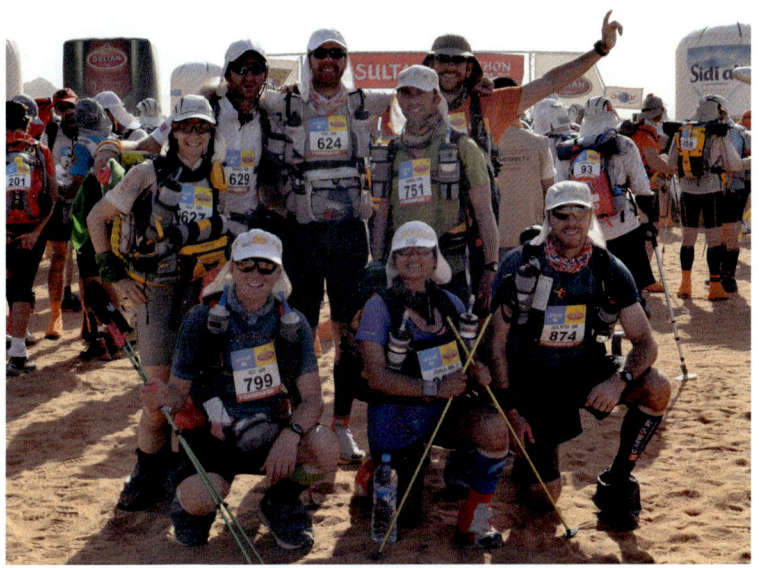

Team picture before stage two of MDS – everyone in tent 110 (I'm front right, Paul is middle of the top row). (Author's own collection)

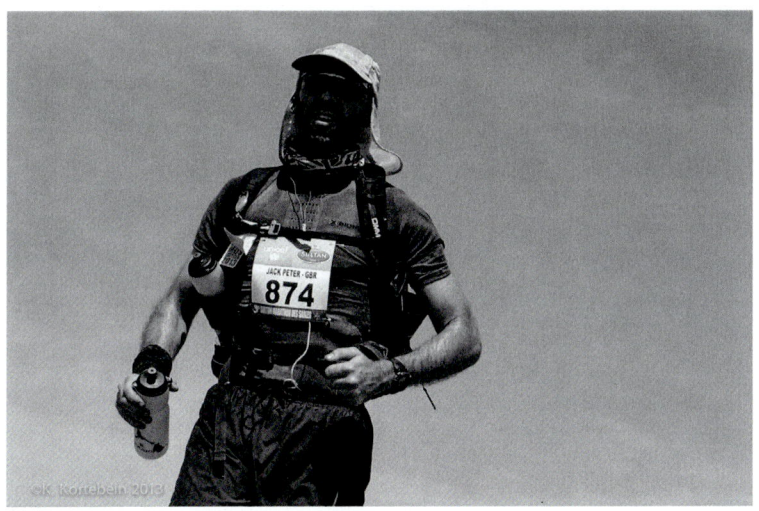

The finishing line in sight at MDS 2013.
(Photo credit: Marathon des Sables)

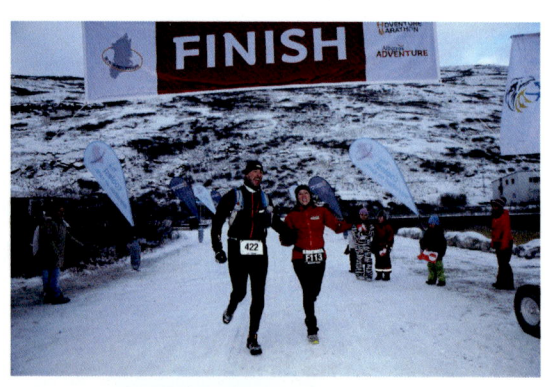

Rachel and me finishing the Polar Circle Marathon in 2014. A wonderful memory. (Photo credit: Albatros Adventure Marathons)

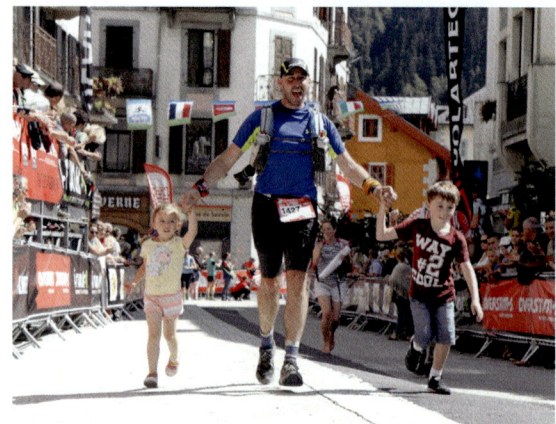

Finishing UTMB in 2014 with the family in Chamonix. My favourite running picture. (Author's own collection)

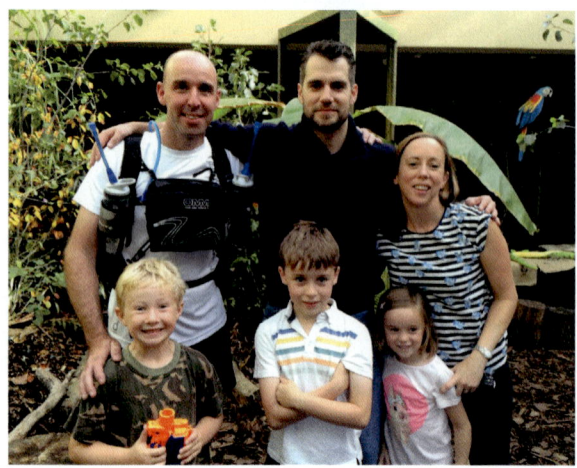

The Wrights meeting Henry Cavill in 2015, along with Steve's son, Evan. (Author's own collection)

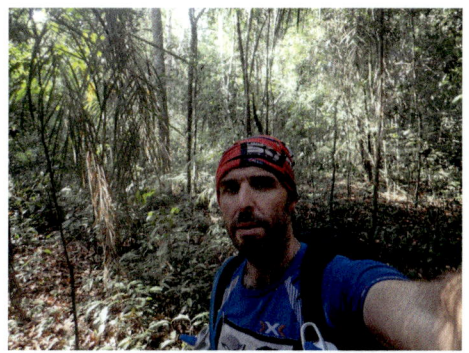

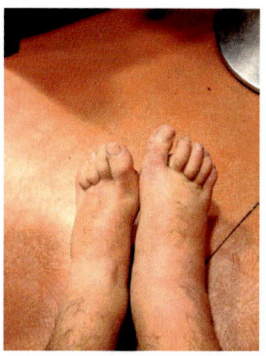

Scared in the jungle after a very close encounter with a jaguar. (Author's own collection)

The state of my feet after the Jungle Marathon. (Author's own collection)

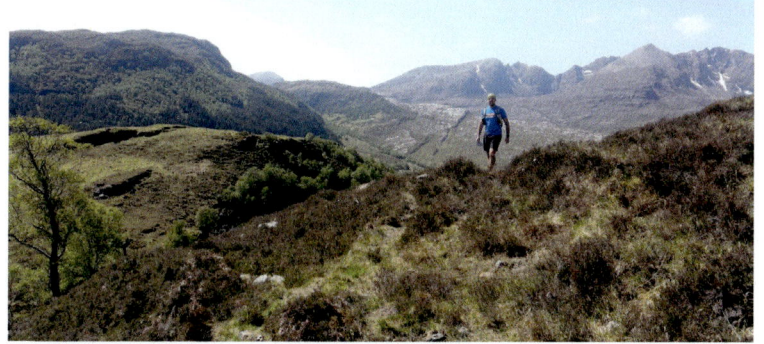

Breathtaking scenery throughout Cape Wrath in 2016. (Author's own collection)

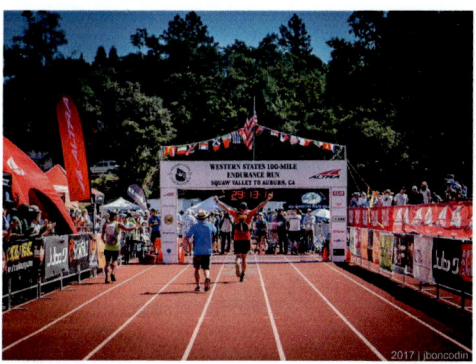

Finishing the Western States 100 in the 'Golden Hour'. Michael Li (my support crew) is filming the moment on my far left. (Author's own collection)

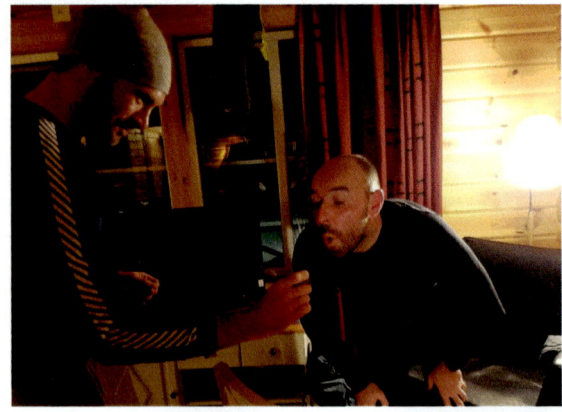

Simon Davies wishing me a happy birthday at the Ice Ultra. (Author's own collection)

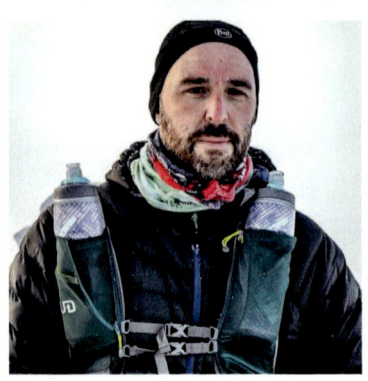

Feeling slightly chilly in the Ice Ultra on day two as temperatures reached -45°C.

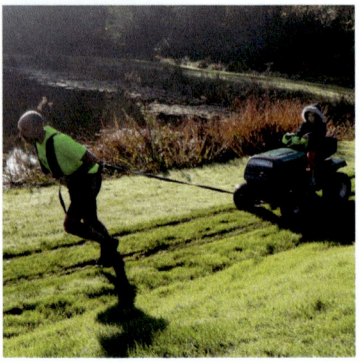

Practising for the Marathon Car Pull in 2019 at my parents' house. My enthusiastic daughter helping also. (Author's own collection)

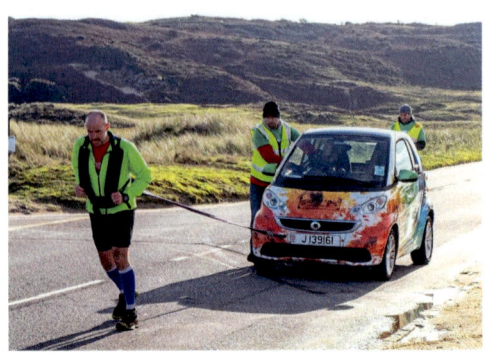

Grimacing at the halfway point of the Marathon Car Pull in 2019. My good friend, Stuart, is helping to steer the car. (Author's own collection)

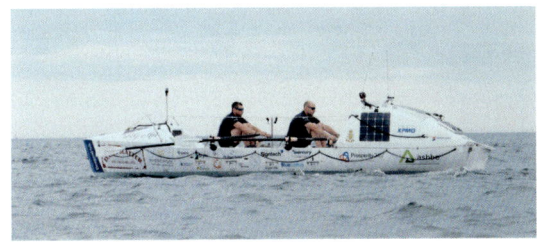

Steve and I getting our qualifying hours in on our home island of Jersey. (Photo credit: Matt Sharp)

The official pre-race team shot, taken a couple of days before the start of the Talisker Whisky Atlantic Challenge. (Photo credit: World's Toughest Row)

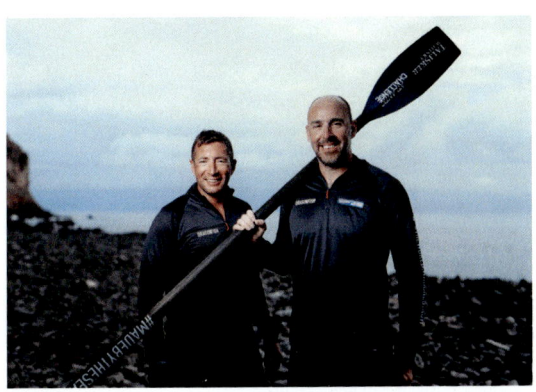

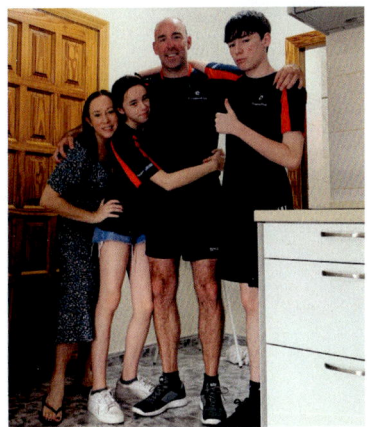

With Rachel and the kids just before I left the apartment on 12 December. I made this my screensaver and it kept me going throughout my 54 days at sea. (Author's own collection)

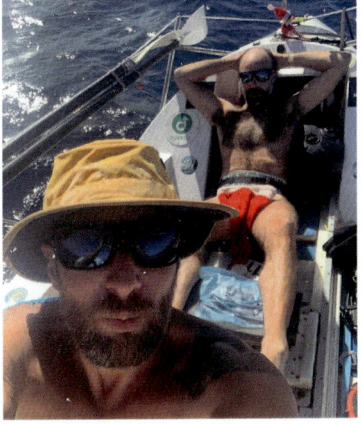

A more relaxing moment on the row. I think I still have the Santa hat somewhere. (Author's own collection)

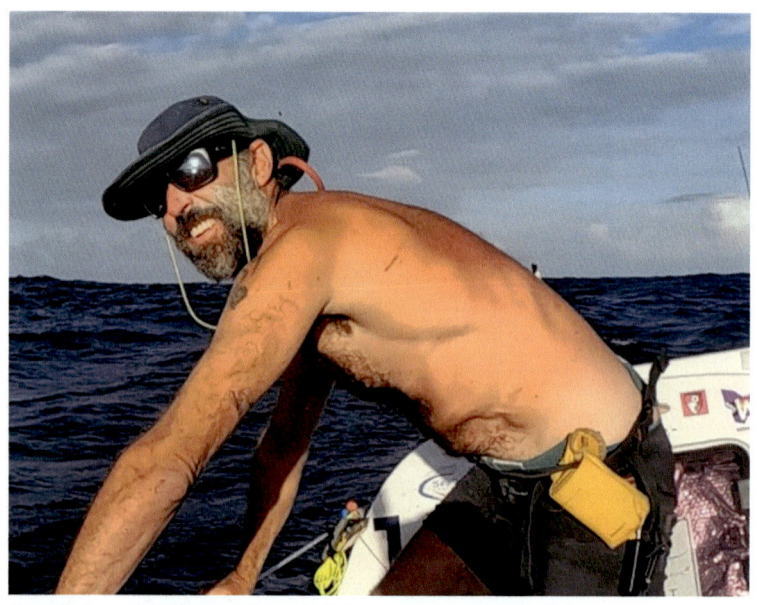

Land ahoy! My first sighting of Antigua on our 52nd day at sea. (Author's own collection)

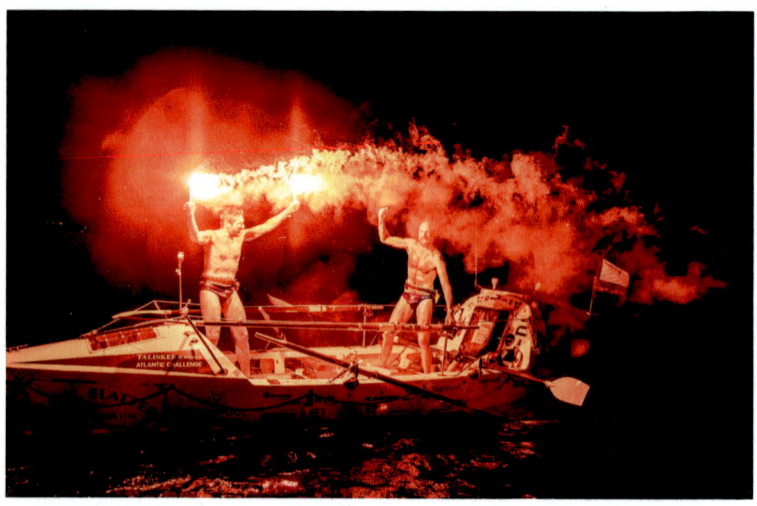

Steve holding the flares and me punching the air at the race's finish. (Photo credit: World's Toughest Row)

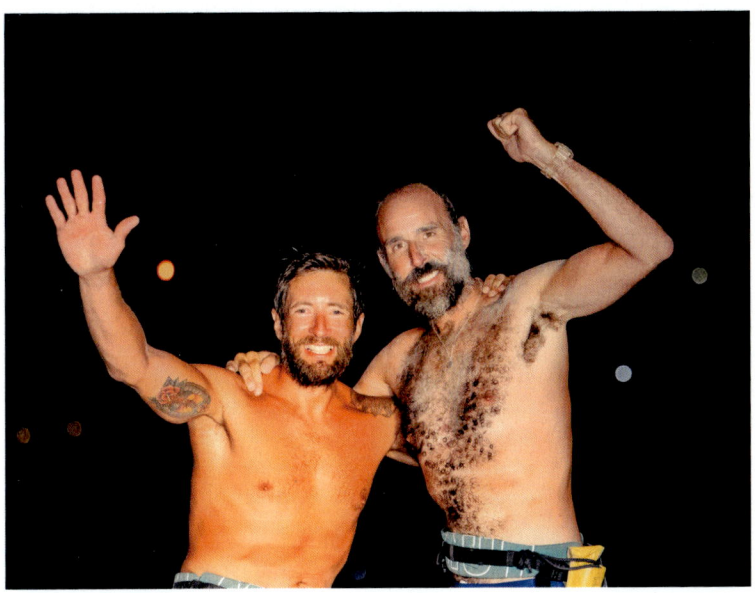

Brothers in arms. Steve somehow managing to make me look very pasty on arrival into Antigua. (Photo credit: World's Toughest Row)

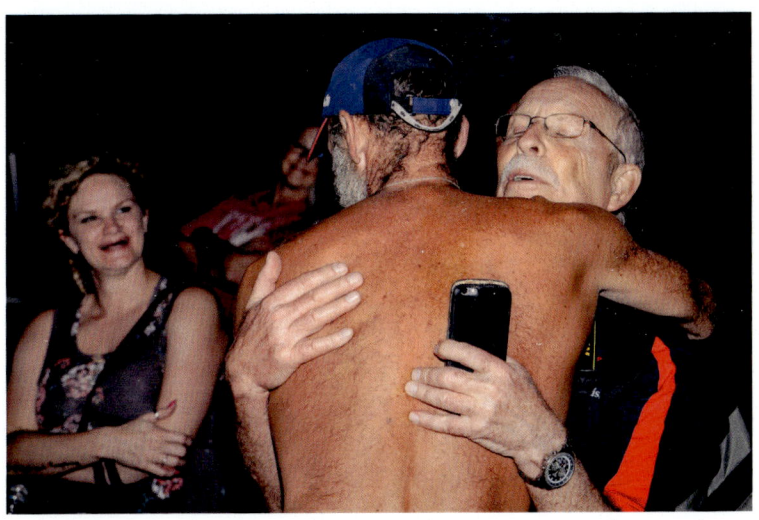

A warm embrace with my Dad on arrival into Antigua. (Photo credit: World's Toughest Row)

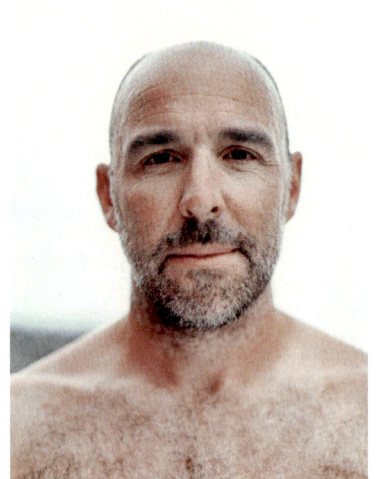
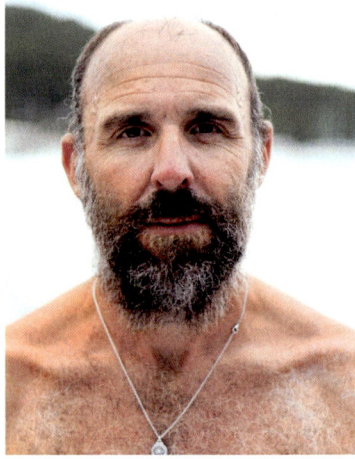

The official before and after shots taken by Atlantic Campaigns. Good job Steve didn't let me shave. (Photo credit: World's Toughest Row)

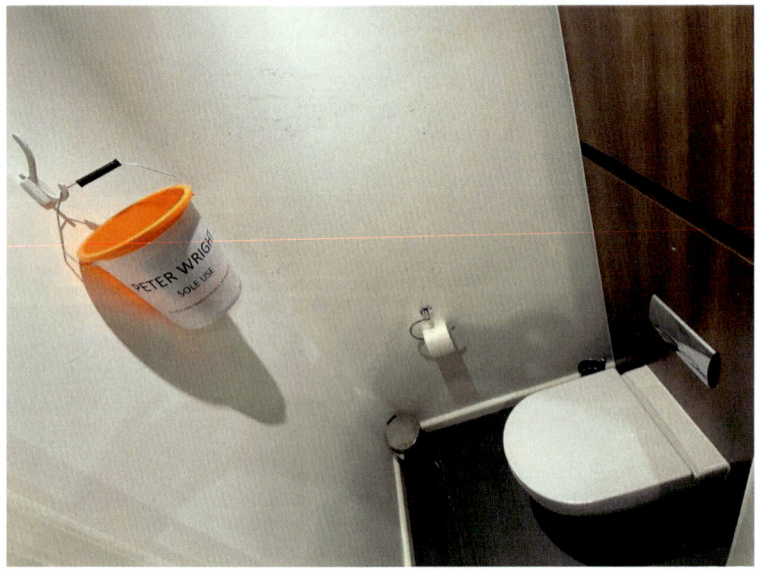

My work colleagues kindly helping me acclimatise to life back on land. (Author's own collection)

Interlude 9

THINGS WERE going well. After a couple of weeks at sea, we were still a long way from Robin Knox-Johnston territory, but were feeling comfortable. We'd established a routine; we were in the lead, and we were happy. We had regular contact with home, we'd had a bit of an argument/ discussion about our strengths and weaknesses, and put better action plans in place to deal with the incoming bad weather that would really test our nerves and our boat-handling skills.

This bad weather would ultimately see us having to abandon the idea of rowing and hunker down in the cabin for the better part of four days.

This became a very low point for me, and, I'm sure, Pete too, although he seemed to deal with it better. The winds and waves had picked up, so we couldn't row without a big risk of capsize. We deployed our drogue and decided to wait it out. This led to two options: wait outside while getting drenched every few seconds and being able to witness each terrifying wave and wondering if it would be the one to roll us and potentially sink us, or stay in the swelteringly hot and airless cabin, wishing the days away and hoping the depression would fizzle out.

We'd swap regularly due to boredom, discomfort and not having enough space inside. During the night, we'd both try to sleep inside, but with two naked (because of the heat) adults there wasn't a lot of room to move around, and things quickly became sweaty and sticky.

Our sores became worse as the friction from our coarse boat mattress rubbed at any contact points – shoulder blades, hips, heels, bums. I could go on forever, but it was just a miserable, airless, claustrophobic place to be, and no amount of games, jokes or iPad movies would help.

During one particularly long and restless night in the sweat box, I woke to the feeling of something touching my bare arse. Obviously, it was Pete, but he was asleep and we were sleeping top to toe and back to back. Our arses came together in a sweaty and puss-ridden mess. I was alarmed. Scared, even. Maybe I found it funny. What should I do? Should I wake him? I couldn't go anywhere. Rolling away wasn't an option, and I certainly wasn't going to turn around. It seemed that a bit of arse-to-arse contact was the best idea of a bad bunch, so I thought, 'Bollocks, I'll just lean against him and get some rest.'

The fact that we'd given up our lead just compounded the frustrations. Things could only get better, surely.

Steve Hayes

Chapter 10

Brave hurt

THE CAPE Wrath Ultra was an event that I'd heard about a few years previously. Taking place over eight days across 400km of spectacular Highland scenery from Fort William all the way to the titular mount, it immediately grabbed my attention. The thought of running this trail, situated in one of the most beautiful places in the world, was an opportunity that I wasn't going to let pass by – not to mention that 2016 was to be the maiden voyage of the event.

The brainchild of race director Shane Ohly, I was familiar with the setup of his races, having tackled Dragon's Back the previous year (a DNF, but still a valuable learning curve). Taking place 88 per cent on trail, I knew that organisation, navigational awareness, training and kit choices would be crucial. I'd spent quite some time practising my navigation prior to this event, so was fairly confident with a map in my hand. In addition, I ensured that I downloaded the daily GPX tracks to my handheld Garmin so that there was an adequate backup plan.

One side-effect of living in Jersey is that the travel routes are always varied, and so it proved here: Jersey to

Southampton; to Glasgow and, finally, Fort William. Along the way, I came across various faces both new and familiar: first was Jon Gittins, who I met while we were competing in the Polar Circle Marathon, and Kirsten Ejlscov Jensen from Denmark, who we chatted with about our various running challenges and future aspirations while on the train to Fort William. Another reunion was had with Gwyn Stokes during the briefing – last seen in vastly less favourable circumstances, as we were both carted off in the back of a van at the Spine. We both hoped that this time would be different!

During the registration process, our photos were taken by the highly talented Ian Corless. Mine resulted in me looking slightly sinister and more than a bit evil, which my mates back home were keen to remind me of in my final dose of social media before the event!

Day 1: Fort William to Glenfinnan. Distance 37km, Height Gain 500m

Heralded by a bagpiper, the race began with a 10km road stretch along the shores of Loch Linnhe. I wanted to ease into things, so started with a steady jog. This would be a relatively short and simple day compared to what was to come, and presented an opportunity to take in all the scenery, as well as to put my navigation skills into practice – something Jersey, with its distinct lack of endless wilderness, doesn't really provide.

There was a really good vibe among the competitors, and it's always fun early on in events getting to know people. I remember coming across a guy who I thought had entered the wrong event on account of his rucksack size (it had to weigh over 15kg).

'Which race have you entered, mate?' I asked with a slightly mischievous smile. He told me that it had been his dream to explore this part of Scotland, and he wanted to capture as much quality imagery as he could en route.

As it turned out, this guy, Frank Tschöpe, from Germany, was carrying all of his photography equipment. Dedicated to his profession, he proved to be an absolute legend for getting some amazing shots while completing the event in a very respectable time.

Afterwards came some equally runnable double track westbound towards Conaglen estate. The double tracks eventually gave way to more challenging terrain in the form of wet and muddy paths by the mountain of Sgorr Craobh. I'd decided to test the waters with my New Balance Leadvilles, which are both comfy on trails and pretty good on the road. However, these were proving hard work in the wet conditions, and I experienced several slides and stumbles, particularly over wet rock. I knew I'd be switching to my grippy and equally comfortable Salomon Speedcross trainers for the subsequent days.

The day finished with a nice run descending into Glenfinnan and camp for the day. This was located near the viaduct that the Hogwarts Express is seen on in the *Harry Potter* films, so I made sure a few pictures were taken to share with my son Josh, who was mad about the films at the time.

Before I went to sleep, I checked the map and the distance of the subsequent days' routes. It really hit home what I'd let myself in for. This was going to be a massive challenge and hopefully an adventure of a lifetime.

Day 2: Glenfinnan to Kinloch Hourn. Distance 57km, Height Gain 1,800m

The day began with the breakfast of champions: baked beans, egg and bread – as it would be every day for the entire course. I'm a lifelong baked bean addict, but this event severely tested that addiction.

Sadly, before setting off, I noticed that my tent mate, Lee Walker, was looking underprepared.

'I'm pretty sure it's plantar fasciitis,' he said grimly. 'My race is over.' I really felt for him, since he'd looked so strong on day one, and had been buzzing when I first met him at the race briefing. It was another reminder of how tough things could get, and how anything can suddenly impact your race in a negative way.

After the short briefing from Shane – another standard daily procedure – we set off.

I couldn't put my finger on it, but I felt heavy-legged from the off. Nevertheless, I soon got into a steady running pattern, and the day passed by in a blur of endurance and exhaustion. One of the lesser-trodden parts of the route, the terrain was incredibly strength-sapping, with plenty of short and sharp climbs. I'd damaged a tendon in the Jungle Marathon the previous year, and all the sinking and twisting was playing havoc with it.

A couple of hours later, I received a pleasant surprise. Lee came running past with a massive grin on his face. As it turned out, he'd had a chat with Marcus Scotney, who had been coaching him for this event. Marcus applied Kinesio tape to relieve the pressure and pain. This epitomised the sort of guy that Marcus – the eventual event winner by a country mile – is. Whenever I saw him run past me – which occurred early on each day – he'd always be smiling and giving out encouragement. He was exactly the same in camp as the competitors finished each day's stage. Marcus is, without doubt, one of the nicest guys I've met on the ultrarunning circuit.

As Jon Gittins (my travel companion for this event, who I'd met at the Polar Circle Marathon, quickly becoming good friends) and I trudged across the Carnach Estuary, I was sinking all over the place, with my ankles and limbs taking a battering, no doubt giving Stu Smith, who was part of the race crew, a right old laugh.

As I approached checkpoint two, a very jolly Stu shouted out, 'You struggling a little there, Pete?' all the while sporting a mischievous grin. Stu is very much like Papa Smurf in appearance, and just as jolly. There are always plenty of laughs when he's around. I managed a grimace in response – to say I was struggling was not an understatement.

Beyond checkpoint two, we had a period of respite as we travelled alongside the river. This was much needed, since my legs had felt significantly worked from the last stretch, and I needed to get some life back in them. I knew we needed to look out for what can only be described as a bastard of a climb at a turning point on the river, which at this point was filling me with dread. I was absolutely blowing out of my backside as I lumbered up.

Some dark thoughts were entering my head: *Do I have it in me to complete this?* It just wasn't happening! The others just told me not to overthink it, play the long game, put one foot in front of the other, look around and take comfort in the surroundings. I decided to pay more attention to that voice.

With multiday events, it can sometimes take a little while for your body to adjust to what you're putting it through – my transition from office worker to busting out 400km was proving this to be the case. That said, after a couple of days, it starts to happen. As long as the mind remains strong and focused, the body will generally follow.

Jon and I finished in around 12 hours – far longer than I'd wanted, and resulting in me feeling far more knackered than I was hoping for. And 12 hours 'out on the hill' meant there would be less time to relax and recover at camp. I was conscious that there was a very tough day to follow, and there wasn't a whole lot of time to recover. However, I'd learned some lessons from my DNF at Dragon's Back from an administrative perspective, and had carefully prepared separate dry bags, which consisted of the kit and supplies I'd need for each day's stage, so this was one less thing to think about.

It was good to chat with the others about the day's events. Mick Cooper, one of my tent mates, was a complete gentleman, on hand with a heavenly cup of tea. Jacquie, Mick's wife, was part of the support crew, and she was equally lovely. Such kind gestures in a challenge mean a lot, and there were plenty of people like Mick and Jacquie in the Cape Wrath family.

Day 3: Kinloch Hourn to Achnashellach. Distance 68km, Height Gain 2,400m

Jon and I started at a decent pace, despite not having slept well at all, and made a steady climb over Bealach

Coire Mhalagain. It was during this that we met one of our companions, Scott Clarke, who led the charge on the descent to Kintail & Morvich, full of ankle-twisting tussocks and boggy ground, which by now I was getting very used to – my ankles and tendons were feeling very elastic. Despite this, I was feeling a lot better. Scott also mentioned that there was potentially a place to grab a coke, which gave me a monumental lift.

Sure enough, we found a small restaurant, and Scott delivered. Heaven in a can, it lifted our spirits immediately. We carried on along a road, before once again hitting some mixed terrain. We were now part of a group of six or seven, heading inland to pass the Falls of Glomach. As we approached the descent, we arrived at the edge of a gorge, to be met by some confusion and differing opinions on which path to take.

'I've got a suspicion that this might not be the route,' I helpfully pointed out as we started descending an ankle-breaker of a path. The adjustment was made, and soon enough we began our correct descent to Loch Leitreach, and much kinder terrain at Carnach. Tiredness was really creeping in, but I was in good spirits.

These were reduced slightly when I came across Lee. He hadn't been able to keep food down, and had to withdraw. I found him sitting on a tree stump looking pretty fatigued.

'I'll take this as decent training for next year,' he said. Sometimes, it just isn't your day or race. However, he did carry on after this day, completing some other stages, and I never saw him without a smile on his face.

There were many people like him, and I admired each of them for their spirit and attitude.

We continued in a small group, and came across Simon Hodson, who was having a tough day, as an old injury was coming back to haunt him, prompting him to do his best with some DIY repairs. Simon was a strong-looking lad who liked to challenge himself, but I could see that he was in a lot of pain. He looked at me and said one word: 'Brutal.' We had a quick chat, and I checked he was okay to keep moving – he reassured me that he was. I think Simon did complete this day, but had to rest up on day four before continuing.

The magnitude of the day was starting to sink in as we once again hit rougher ground after Loch Cruoshie. This part was quite fun, and involved jumping over bogs and puddles, with a high likelihood of sinking to your waist, à la *Vicar of Dibley*.

After what seemed like the longest 2km ever, we hit the wire bridge, which I'd really been looking forward to. Getting across this with stiff, Cyberman-type legs was a laugh a minute. Beyond this was a nice, runnable trail alongside a stunning, picturesque loch. The last few miles, for me, summarised what was so brilliant about this event – you were never far away from natural beauty. All that lay between us and the day's finish was one beast of a climb, a cold, windswept summit, and a rather painful descent into camp.

I enjoyed the climb, which was in a nice marching pattern, accompanied by Scott and Stevie Clare. I'd met Stevie at certain times on the previous two days, and we'd also go on to both complete Dragon's Back a few years later. She was in a world of pain, like all of us, but I was being very generous, handing out sweets and generally being really positive. I enjoyed Stevie's company, and it was always quite refreshing having a conversation with her.

At the top of this climb, for the only time in the event, I felt very cold due to the wind chill, so it was a case of getting through the next few hundred metres and descending to lower ground as soon as possible. We could see camp, but it took an age to get there. Eventually, the rugged terrain gave way to forest trail. Bounding through the forest, knowing that camp was imminent, was brilliant.

The day's course took me 15 hours, with Jon coming in a short while later. It looked like the last two days had taken a lot out of him. We'd been in darkness for the final couple of hours of this stage, and the longer the day meant less time for recovery. Thankfully, I'd put a great deal of effort in organising my drop bag, and knew exactly where everything was located for the following day's stage.

Unfortunately, I didn't see Scott beyond this day. I heard later that he'd had to pull out on account of his blister issues, which was a real shame. It really hammered home just how unpredictable these events are, and how you should take nothing for granted and enjoy it while you can.

Day 4: Achnashellach to Kinlochewe. Distance 35km, Height Gain 1,400m

I had it in my head that this would be the 'easy' day, since the distance was considerably less than the previous two days. It didn't turn out that way at all. I started off with Jon, and soon enough we began a long, steady climb. I was moving at a very different speed to Jon, waiting at frequent intervals during the climb for him to catch up. Upon reaching the top, I waited five minutes or so, and with no sign, I pushed on, really hoping he'd catch up.

Ultimately, you need to run your own race. It's not easy being the leader who waits, or the follower who is most likely pushing themselves too hard in order to keep up. I've experienced both scenarios, but did feel guilty for pushing on.

I maintained decent progress, and made checkpoint one with ease, feeling really positive about the day. After being on my own for some time, I joined up with Stuart Secker and Louise Watson. I'd not properly met either until this point, so it was a case of making introductions and exchanging notes about our experiences to date. We all agreed that days two and three had been tough.

I've kept in touch with Stuart, who later managed to secure entry to Western States the year after me. I was therefore able to make introductions to Michael Li, who ended up acting as his support crew, just as he'd done for me.

We ascended to Loch Coire Mhic Fhearchair, and were greeted with some absolutely stunning scenery. The place was breathtaking, and we all took some time to admire its natural beauty.

After leaving the loch, we headed east. I was now in the company of Angus McArthur and Phil Humphries. As with Stuart and Louise, I hadn't met either until this point, so it was a case of swift introductions and then collaborative problem-solving regarding the route ahead. I enjoyed meeting up with different people along the way, and both guys were very laid-back and good company.

Unfortunately, although we found ourselves on the right bearing, we were a lot higher than we should have been, and the longer we continued the harder it would be to drop down. As it was, we were already 250m too high, and we could see where we needed to be after spotting the trail below. The subsequent descent was precarious, to say the least, and it was achieved any way we could, with plenty of time on the backside. The hidden rocks, potholes and tussocks weren't appreciated. Still, it was nice to get a bumpy massage on the buttocks.

As the three of us descended, we spotted other runners moving east below us on the correct path, so we got down as quickly as we could and all moved forwards together in a group of six. Once on the path, I was unable to maintain the pace of the others and figured that, with plenty of time on my side, I'd take a slow plod to the finish and save some energy for day five.

Camp was a welcome sight, and it was early afternoon, so relatively early compared to the previous two days. This was great, since I actually had some time to recover. I retrieved my drop bag and got myself sorted out. This involved sitting in the blazing sunshine on a deckchair with my feet in a washing-up bowl of cold, clean water. Heavenly!

An hour later, I was probably on my third portion of chips when I saw Jon come through. Initial thoughts were positive, but then I heard his tone of voice, which suggested otherwise. 'I've been disqualified,' he told

Shane. It turned out he'd headed north six miles instead of east shortly after the waterfall, and had been picked up on the main road – well off the map. I think there had been an option to continue along a very busy road with a time penalty, but he decided against this. However, soon enough and after a phone conversation with his wife, he was his usual positive self, and decided to stick around and enjoy some of the other days.

The evening was spent with a nice meal in the local pub, which was an absolute luxury, and I was feeling well and truly recharged. I avoided beer, though – I was saving that for when I completed the event.

Day 5: Kinlochewe to Inverlael. Distance 44km, Height Gain 1,400m

Jon's feet were very swollen, so it was beneficial that he was skipping today's stage. Off the back of never having run an ultra, he'd carved out around 125 miles in four days – an incredible achievement.

It was easy to pick up on some conversations from other tents, and I could frequently hear Gilliam Boogerd's infectious, high-pitched laugh above everything else. Usually, he'd be ripping the piss out of one of his tent mates, and it was amusing to overhear his tactics for reeling them in during a conversation and dealing a hammer piss-take blow. I think it was the transition of his calm Dutch accent to hysterical laughter that always put a smile on my face when I overheard him at work. I greatly enjoyed his company, and shared a fair few beers with him at the afterparty.

The other thing I remember about Gilliam was the state of his feet – they'd got progressively worse throughout the event, and he was particularly susceptible to blisters. I remember him laughing and saying to me, 'I probably won't be able to go into work for weeks with the state of these. My wife's going to kill me.' Even so, he did go on to complete the race, with a good time, considering what he went through.

This stage started following a nice, easy track with Louise Watson. Soon enough, we began climbing, maintaining a steady pace in convoy. From here, we headed inland through Bealach na Croise, now off-track. The ground was rough and full of tussocks, while very boggy in places. The scenery was once again mind-blowing – at one point we saw a dozen wild deer run by.

After navigating this terrain, we found another path and headed north alongside Loch an Nid. For a while, I jogged along without a care in the world. Towards the end of the loch, I began a steady ascent towards checkpoint one.

It was during this that I came across Darren Grigas, who was in some degree of pain with a shin injury. Nevertheless, he was grinning away. It wasn't going to stop him. From memory, when I came across him, he was filming tadpoles with his GoPro. Each to their own.

I spent a little time in Darren's company as we moved along through a scenic part of the trail. We compared notes about the MDS, where he shared a tent with Rory Coleman (my MDS mentor) and Sir Ranulph Fiennes. He told me just how determined Sir Ranulph was, and how much respect he had for him. In Darren's words, 'At 71 years old, he was out there much longer than us nippers, and therefore cooking twice as long.'

Slightly further on, Jonathan Douglass had noticed that Darren was in some pain as he hobbled along with his painful shin, and lent him one of his walking poles. It was a great gesture, and typified the growing camaraderie between all the competitors. While people are technically competing against each other, it doesn't often feel that way; the atmosphere was more of a 'we're all in this together' kind of thing. It was one of the many factors that made events like this so uniquely welcoming.

I moved on alone to descend on mostly runnable trail. The day had been hot, showing no signs of cooling down. So far, it had been a rather unique week of weather in western Scotland – not a drop of rain, and blue sky with the sun shining. I found the descent very painful, since by now the knees and quads were feeling overworked. However, with a face that probably looked rather constipated, I was down quickly enough. The last half-mile was spent on a flat road running into camp at an enjoyable pace. I was given a choc ice by one of the race crew – officially the best choc ice ever!

The last two days had been very uplifting in terms of scenery (plenty of rolling hills, blue skies and untouched natural beauty – the backdrops in *The Lord of the Rings* film trilogy came to mind) and having plenty of time at camp to chill out and recover. These two days were a masterstroke by Shane and the team, and afforded everyone the chance to recharge. The next two days, at 45 and 38 miles, respectively, were going to be a huge test, but my mind was positive and raring to go.

Day 6: Inverlael to Inchnadamph. Distance 72km, Height Gain 1,400m

I woke with an intense pain on my lower left shin, noticing swelling, but no bruising. This was slightly worrying with 100 miles to go, but there were plenty of others in the same boat.

This was never going to be a walk in the park. Jon was also well rested, and on the start line to get day six done.

'Back in the game,' he said. 'I'll give you a piggyback if you like?'

It was great to have his company again. The day started with a steady winding trail up through a forest with good underfoot terrain. Once again, I was really enjoying the climbing, and maintaining a strong pace. It was clear that today was going to be a very hot day. I was somewhat more apprehensive about the descents on account of my now-painful shin.

With the first mountain section complete, we continued on to Glen Douchary, where the terrain became substantially less enjoyable. The tussocks, bog and rough, unpredictable ground were fast becoming my nemesis, with ankles twisting and knees jarring at frequent intervals. To maintain a degree of sanity, I started keeping score between the two, which took my mind off it a little.

Around this time, the shin pain was becoming really intense and the swelling greater. My calf guard was also causing me discomfort by compressing it, so I rolled that down to alleviate some pressure. The descents were particularly harsh – it felt like a chisel was knocking against my shin. After what seemed like an eternity, we began a more enjoyable ascent on track and ultimately bound to checkpoint one.

We maintained steady progress along the path and, at Allt Rugaidh Mhor, I'd been keeping an eye out for a right-hand path, since there was a risk we could overshoot this. Ultimately, we did anyway by about 50m, but after taking a grid reference, realised our error and tracked back to find the path.

There was now a nice, runnable route to Loch Ailsh, but my shin had me in so much pain that I could only manage a fast walk. This was greatly frustrating, since there were so many runnable parts at this point.

Eventually, we reached the loch, and began a northerly bearing, which was leading to the finish. There was some distance still to cover, and it would be slow going. The ground became tougher underfoot, and my legs felt like they had nothing left. It had been a long day, with constant high temperatures. I was the most tired and low I'd been during the event.

After what felt like a very long death march, we found ourselves in a group of six, and tackled the last part of the course. This involved climbing to higher ground by the gorge and finding the path for the final descent into camp. Mark Rawlinson and David Rennie were kind enough to let me tag along, and I kept them in sight as we descended. I explained that I was pretty much done in.

'Just follow us and do what we do. We won't leave you behind,' said David. Even though I couldn't handle conversation at this point, it was just nice to have some supportive company. For me, the end couldn't come quickly enough on account of the shin pain. That said, I was delighted with my time, and gave myself a big pat on the back.

On arrival in camp, I had a quick chat with the medic about the pain, and got my feet and shin into a bucket of loch water.

'On a scale of 1–10, how painful?' asked the medic.

'Um, 9.5,' I replied.

'Well, you've got 0.5 to play with then,' he replied, before reassuring me that ice, painkillers and a good feed would do me the world of good.

What followed was one of the most relaxing experiences of the event: my feet were cooling off, I had a cold can of coke, and I was reading messages from my wife and kids.

'Daddy, Mummy says you have run 300 miles and you are our superhero. We're telling all our friends at school tomorrow,' read one from Josh. Cue watery eyes and a wobbly lip while looking ahead at a beautiful loch. Could life really get any better?

Jon was buzzing when he came in 30 minutes later, and rightly so. He'd exorcised the demons of two days previous, and done an amazing job. His feet were badly swollen, and he'd really had to dig deep. We spent a couple of hours down the pub, where the landlord gave me a bag of ice for my shin. What I really wanted was a heavenly pint of milk, and the landlord duly obliged. Darren, who later joined us, was easily corrupted to the milk gang, as were a few other competitors. Record pints of milk were served on that day.

Day 7: Inchnadamph to Kinlochbervie. Distance 61km, Height Gain 1,600m

If I was able to complete this day, I knew the event was in the bag, given the relatively shorter distance on day eight. Therefore, I left camp on my own at 7am, feeling very motivated, with the simple mantra of 'one foot in front of the other, repeat'. My tent mate from the MDS, Gordon Marshall, had put that little saying in my head.

I started off very well, and took the first long and steady ascent strongly. After this, I hit some more challenging terrain, passing the spectacular Eas a' Chual Aluinn – Britain's highest waterfall. What followed was a horrible stretch as I headed to Loch Beag and east along the shore. It was slow going, my ankles and knees going every direction possible. I was in some pain, solely focused on the bridge at the end of the loch, sincerely hoping that west along the opposite side would be easier.

Thankfully, it was. It had been some time since I'd run, so it was difficult to forge a rhythm. Eventually, I got going towards the waterfall at Malde Burn, so much so that I overshot my planned turning. I found myself on another steep and steady climb, again surrounded by spectacular views of the waterfalls, followed by Loch a Leathaid Bhuain. After my previous error, I was mindful to keep an eye out for the north-west path to Ben Dreavie.

I found myself on my own among lots of small lochs and in complete tranquillity. It was quite a special moment for me, so I decided it was time for lunch – a trusty pepperoni wrap. I'd just about finished when Angus and Mark came by, so I gladly joined their company for the next stretch. This started with a trek across rougher ground and required careful navigation, ultimately leading to a path that descended into checkpoint one. I was proving to be very slow on the more technical descents, and found that the others were moving faster than me. However, with decent progress being made, I ran and walked into checkpoint one.

Hitting checkpoint one was important, since it meant only 10–12km of the rough stuff before joining the road to the finish. Beyond here was a good path to follow, and I was able to keep Mark in my sights. There was a slightly tricky navigational part to reach the path along Loch a'Garbh-bhaid Mòr, but I used my GPS to stay on track.

I found the path, hoping for a nice coast to the road. However, it was anything but – I found it really hard to stay on my feet, and once again I was in a lot of pain. I came across Alex Reilly, who looked as fatigued as me. However, there were no complaints from either of us, being surrounded by such natural beauty.

I pushed on to checkpoint two with the sole mission of getting a coke in for Alex and me, since I knew there was a pub. After receiving quite a few weird looks at the bar as we strolled in (apparently there weren't too many patrons decked out in compressed running gear), I accomplished my mission – along with some salted crisps – before we headed off on the final road section.

This stretch was mostly runnable, although my legs felt like anything but running. It was funny: while on the nasty stretch of trail we'd been on before, I was longing for something flat, but now I was here it was equally painful, with a hard road surface playing havoc with my shin.

Alex ran on ahead as the caffeine took effect, and I jogged on behind, slowly picking up the pace as the painkillers I'd wolfed down with my coke started to kick in.

Just before the end of the stage, I passed John Minta. I'd seen John at the end of day six, and he looked in a bad way, carrying what looked to be a serious injury. I'd also observed him nailing some really technical terrain in previous stages. This guy was hard as nails, and he'd done amazingly well to get today done in the time he had. I spent some time with him post-event and, as it turned out, he'd gifted his finisher's medal to a fellow competitor who had missed one of the days. It spoke volumes about him as a person.

At the finish, Jon and Mick, both tent mates, were there to see me over the line. I finished off the day giving the feet a well-earned cooling in the loch, and several servings of chips.

Day 8: Kinlochbervie to Cape Wrath. Distance 26km, Height Gain 700m

The route was much shorter today, but after studying the map it was clear that the second half, after Sandwood Bay, would be tougher going. I switched back to the Salomons and was ready to go.

I started with Jon at walking pace while the shin warmed up. Soon enough, we were in a steady running pattern, joined by Mark Keddie and Con Bonner. As we progressed along the first half of the route towards the beach, Mark and I found ourselves moving fairly swiftly and getting into a good running pattern, with Jon and Con not too far behind.

Up until Sandwood Bay, it was fairly easy going, and the actual views of the bay were an uplifting sight.

There seemed little point in running on the energy-sapping sand, so we power-walked across and began to ascend.

With the terrain becoming more challenging, with numerous ascents and descents, my shin was once again on fire. I was now becoming extremely slow on the more technical descents, carefully placing each foot strike and desperately trying to manage the pain – a group of around ten runners easing past me as I struggled on down.

However, today was all about absorbing the final experience, and just after Sithean na h-Iolaireich, Mark and I verified our GPS route. All that was left was to stay on the correct bearing and find the path that led to the lighthouse at Cape Wrath: the finish line. Soon enough we did, and settled into a steady run.

It was amazing to see the lighthouse. The feeling was one of elation; relief that I could give my shin a rest, excitement that I'd be going home to see Rach and the kids, and also a little bit of sadness that the adventure was nearly over. It had been a unique eight days, where I'd really seen western Scotland in its full glory and the weather had completely been onside, with not a drop of rain.

I managed to run in just as the first minibus was leaving with the lead runners of this day's stage. I was able to high-five the windows of the van before crossing the line, and got my picture taken by Ian Corless at the iconic lighthouse.

There was a very small café there, so I grabbed myself a hot chocolate and a bacon roll, and cheered in a few other runners while I waited for the next minibus.

The vast majority of the runners I've mentioned in this chapter completed the race, and those that didn't were unfortunate not to be able to complete one of the eight stages. However, they still stayed as part of the race and completed all others.

The winner, by some distance, was the incredible Marcus Scotney, who had some engine on him and was a very good navigator. Gwynn Stokes stormed back from his previous Spine disappointment, finishing in 11th. Gwynn has gone on to complete many Spine races, which is some feat. My tent mate, a true gentleman, Mick Cooper, finished in 12th.

A couple of things stood out about this race for me. Firstly, it was by far the longest I'd attempted. Secondly, it required the most self-sufficiency in terms of tactics and navigation, and I spent numerous hours on the course on my own, problem-solving, the effect of camaraderie on keeping spirits up, and putting into practice the navigation skills I'd learned in the build-up. I also saw it as a dress rehearsal for a Dragon's Back rematch. Another Shane Ohly event, completing it would give me the confidence to enter again.

There wasn't a huge number of runners in this race, considering the length of the route. There were 95 starters, of which 59 finished – I was 39th.

It was May 2016, three years since my ultra journey had started, and I was in no mood for sitting still. As I sat on the train on the long journey back down south, I reflected on what was coming up next. The following month, I had the Vegan Welsh 3000s, a relatively 'short' 35-mile race, 4,500m of ascent thrown in. The race itself summits all 15 of the Welsh 3,000ft peaks in a linear race encompassing the Snowdon massive, Glyderau and the Carneddau. Let's just say that I was in no way at all recovered from Cape Wrath, which was a month before, but I'd headed up to the event with some friends I'd met at the Jungle Marathon in 2015. I'd anticipated a nice, social run with one of my friends on the day, but he turned his ankle after two miles and was forced to withdraw at the first checkpoint. I therefore had a lonely and painful journey ahead, but I did complete it, more or less in last place, and found all my other friends very drunk at the finish line.

This would be followed be a rematch for the Spine with Andy McDonald in January 2017. We'd both DNFd that in 2016. What could possibly go wrong? With all that in my mind, I drifted off to sleep. Another ultra ticked off!

Interlude 10

AS A physio, we meet new clients every day. We always start with the same format: take the history of the injury, understand the client's aims and goals, formulate the diagnosis and then together devise a plan of how to help the client achieve their goals. Over the years, we've treated everything from the smallest niggle to life-changing injuries. Along the way, we've met some truly exceptional people – Pete is one of these.

When I first met him, Pete was relatively new to running, and looking towards his first marathon. Over the successive years, I'd learn to anticipate his signature move: he'd nonchalantly lean forward in the chair, elbows on his knees, shrug his shoulders and quietly drop into conversation the next big event he had in mind.

Starting off as a relatively new runner with aspirations of completing his first marathon, Pete's journey has evolved into a series of awe-inspiring feats. Once he'd ticked off a marathon, it wasn't long before he was aiming for bigger distances, greater elevation and technically difficult races. His quiet demeanour belies a fierce willpower that has propelled him to conquer ultramarathons such as the MDS, Western States, Dragon's Back and the Jungle Marathon, among others. It's clear that with each challenge, not only did his physical strength grow, but so did his unwavering mindset. It was probably already there, but I hadn't quite seen it.

Upon reflection, it was not too much of a surprise when Pete began to explore other challenges. The fierce will and determination to fundraise for a host of charities such as Macmillan became the norm. I suspect that, knowing Pete, it became his responsibility to do his utmost for the chosen charities.

His transition from running to doing the Christmas 24-hour cycle challenge around the cycle track at Les Quennevais, to undertaking the marathon car pull in 2019, demonstrated a shift towards more diverse and demanding fundraising endeavours. It was during this time that it became apparent that Pete was not merely a weekend warrior, but someone wholly committed to making a difference through his fundraising endeavours.

The revelation of Pete's goal to compete in the World's Toughest Row took everyone by surprise, especially considering that he had no prior experience of rowing. I have a reliable eyewitness report who told me that they were very amusedly observing two lads in a rowing boat in the bay who appeared to be in difficulty – they could neither steer nor coordinate their strokes. At one point, this group were anticipating that they'd need to rescue Pete and Steve, as they feared they wouldn't make it back to shore.

Despite initial challenges and comical observations of his early rowing attempts, his unwavering determination and resilience ultimately led him to success. The mental resilience is not just a phrase; it's important for all activities, from a 5km run and marathon, to an ultramarathon or, indeed, rowing the Atlantic for 54 days. That's true resilience.

Pete is genuinely one of the good guys. Beyond his remarkable physical accomplishments, his humility, self-deprecation, selflessness and compassionate spirit have endeared him to all those who have had the privilege of crossing paths with him. When we think of Pete, we think of the quote from Adam Grant: 'The attitude that helps most with intense stress is not mindfulness. It's hope. In hard times, it's overwhelming to live only in the present. What brings strength is anticipating a brighter future. Resilience lies in remembering that today's burdens may be lighter tomorrow.'

Pete's efforts have raised thousands for charity, making a meaningful impact on the lives of others. We're honoured to be part of his team and to be able to support him achieve his fundraising goals.

Lisa Mann, The Jersey Sports & Spinal Clinic,
Pete's physio

Chapter 11

Setbacks to comebacks

FINALLY, ON 30 December, we were on the move again. This felt good – sure, we were knackered, aching and all the rest of it, but we were finally making some progress. Our boat had experienced everything the ocean could throw at it, and come back stronger. Despite a multitude of equipment failures, we both had a great deal of confidence in the structure and integrity of our boat. After all, it had successfully completed four Atlantic crossings before we purchased it, and now we were beginning to see why.

We'd also been told by the previous owners, prior to the row, that our boat had never suffered a capsize before, and this had given us a reasonable level of assurance before we set out. However, we were mindful that there could always be a first time, while being happy that it had comfortably handled a few days of battery courtesy of the Atlantic.

We were making good progress again on a bearing of 240, and daily mileage was on the increase. However, since 22 December, we'd been without GPS and effectively chartplotter, too. Our water maker went kaput on 17 December, so we'd been using our manual water maker since then. It was a case of 'adapt and overcome' in respect of these two challenges, and we'd established a sound enough routine for dealing with both.

In the absence of GPS, Tim, our weather router, would provide us with a daily bearing to row on, give us regular updates via WhatsApp or satellite phone on our progress, and let us know whether adjustments were needed.

When it came to making water, Steve or I would manually pump during our break from rowing and store as much as we possibly could. We'd also try to prepare in advance all of our daily meals in the morning, so it would just be a case of needing to make water to quench our thirst. On the positive side, we were getting plenty of sunshine, and our batteries were fully charged, which was just as well; we were going to need them.

We were still sobered up by the plight of Fight Oar Die – we'd got to know their crew members, Will, Chad, Nick and Tommy, before the race. American military veterans, they were as tough as they come, but the storm had effectively ended their race. However, they were safe, and that was the most important thing.

Another team, Mr & Mrs Seas, aka Simon and Nina, had been having rudder issues and were down to just a mile a day – at one point, a yacht had to be dispatched to fit them with a replacement rudder. This must have been mentally torturous for them, and it went to show that sometimes you could just be unlucky. The ocean is an unforgiving environment, and even with all the preparation in the world, a bit of bad luck is all it takes.

I'd quickly come to the conclusion that you were never really in full control, and you had to simply accept that and try to make the best decisions that you could. Steve and I couldn't rely on anything apart from each other and our will to complete the challenge. I recall a good quote I've heard about 'the mind being the strongest muscle'. Never was a truer word spoken.

Regardless, we plugged on. After being stuck in the cabin for all that time, we were itching to get going again. While the familiar aches and pains associated with rowing all day and night quickly made their presence acknowledged again, we were once again ramping up the mileage. Salt sores and the associated pain, along with bashed-up shins, were relatively blissful compared to being stuck in the compact sweat box with constant drips of man sweat along with mattress sores.

Steve and I were firmly embracing the fact that we were now able to get back to two hours on and two hours off rowing, our original plan in terms of a system. The sheer misery of the extended confinement within the cabin had really made us appreciate rowing again. Any discomfort completely outweighed the slow suffocation and misery in the cabin.

Even the equipment on our boat seemed to have taken heed of our improved moods and suddenly started working again. By New Year's Day, the water maker was functioning properly again, having imploded in the first week, and the GPS was back online, along with our chartplotter after about a week on the fritz, and the solar panels were fully charged.

The GPS's return was a particular highlight, since we were able to see our speed and mileage from each shift, which meant we could have some fun.

'Four miles an hour,' I could hear Steve roar as he logged an impressive 6.5 miles from his two-hour shift. I was then able to follow up with the same, as good conditions allowed us to gain much-needed momentum.

With the calmer sea state and the fact everything was operational, we set about making as much water as we possibly could and storing it in our various containers and spare bottles. This was to be a tried-and-tested tactic on the rare occasions that the electric water maker became operational, and we devised a system between us where we could get as much water produced as possible, while being mindful of battery usage. Occasionally, there would be air locks, the process of alleviating of which would involve one of us getting in the cramped cabin, lifting the mattress, accessing the water maker via a hatch, and tapping away with the base of a screwdriver to remove the locks.

Inevitably, this happy state of affairs didn't last – the water maker packed in a few days later, forcing us to return to the joy of manual pumping, and the GPS soon followed suit. Like our ancestors before us, we were forced to navigate by manual compass.

Steve was very positive, and would often say things like, 'If the pioneers of old could successfully cross the ocean without all the technology, then we most certainly can.' It was a speech that would generally motivate me and reset the mind to focus on the positives and what was working, as opposed to what wasn't.

Still, we pressed on, sticking to two hours rowing/ two hours off for the first six days of 2023. This was to now be our system moving forwards, and we'd firmly left the one hour on/one hour off system behind us. The previous system, necessary at the time due to the physical pain we were in, wasn't practical or conducive to the efficiency we needed from now on. We were now averaging about 65 nautical miles a day, and managed to regain our lead over a few of the teams that had overtaken us during the fallow period between Christmas and New Year. Despite equipment setbacks, everything was coming together again, and the positivity of good daily mileage was breeding positivity.

This progress took its toll, however. Both of us had picked up painful knee infections by this point – probably due to the amount of crawling we had to do while undertaking our chores, since standing wasn't always possible – which made performing our daily tasks even more arduous than they already were. Living on an ocean-rowing boat, you have to do many tasks that unavoidably involve putting pressure on your knees.

Steve suffered an awful lot worse than me, having to take antibiotics, and his knee really did swell significantly. He'd also managed to pull a muscle in his back, which I think was triggered by the physical exertion we'd expend trying to turn the boat when gusts caught our stern cabin. I don't think it was helped further by his repeated, unsuccessful attempts at fishing. He wasn't having the best time.

'What have you caught for my dinner, matey?' I asked him after one of his stints with the line.

'Sargassum seaweed soup again, my friend,' was the reply.

While the mood had definitely dipped, progress in terms of mileage was at least good. More than ever, we needed to watch each other's backs. Steve, heavily medicated, emerged from the cabin after one of his rest breaks and got back on the oars. I'd decided to sit at the other side of the boat, which was a good thing, as within five minutes he'd been knocked off his rowing seat twice by renegade waves, and was clearly in a lot of pain. This prompted me to say, 'Get back in the cabin and rest up a bit more, and maybe do a longer shift later on.'

He looked groggy, and not at all enthusiastic about my suggestion, but out of a sense of duty he was trying to wave me away and continue at the oars. I wasn't accepting any fightback on this, though. At this point in time, I felt in better shape than Steve, but knew full well that my time would come, and that Steve would gladly repay the favour. This is what it was all about: we really did need to have each other's back and find ways of getting the best out of each other.

Within two minutes of him getting back in the cabin, I could hear a gentle snoring from within. Good deed done, I duly cracked on with my shift.

The lack of GPS meant that we'd have to be extra vigilant when looking out for other vessels, as was highlighted by a particularly scary incident a couple of days later.

Not being able to conclusively navigate where we were going wasn't the only issue; with GPS down, there was also the worrying prospect that we might not be showing up on the AIS (Automatic Identification System), which ships use to keep track of everyone else in the ocean. The AIS system takes into account all the directions that various vessels are heading in, and will set off an alarm in the boat if the two vessels are on a collision course. This is especially important for small boats like us – we're not going to be the easiest to spot, so it's vital for keeping us safe.

This got hammered home sooner than we thought. During one morning shift, we looked up to see a tanker in our line of sight. Both of us were concerned that, before long, it would be bearing down on us, and there would be a collision risk.

Our instruments hadn't given us any alarm warning that we were on a collision course, and our GPS wasn't working, as usual, but we trusted our eyes and weren't taking any chances. We hadn't really had a chance to practise this exercise, since during our training rows our GPS and chartplotter had been fully operational, making it fairly straightforward in terms of navigating boat traffic.

With the tanker slowly becoming larger, we were both fairly calm in our approach to the situation we were in, but equally terrified of the worst-case outcome.

'I'm going to take a bearing between us and that tanker, and do the same again in a couple of minutes,' I said. The idea here was that if it stayed constant, it would be a clear indicator of whether we could be in trouble. Meanwhile, Steve was having a go at trying to contact the boat itself via VHF, but with little success. No response was received – this heightened our fear that the vessel could be on autopilot.

We could almost imagine a scene with the tanker's pilot merrily snoring, with his feet up, but dearly hoped that this wouldn't be the case. The white flares had also been retrieved from the bow cabin in the event that we'd need to escalate our warning as much as we could.

Since I was taking a bearing off our manual compass in bumpy conditions, the results were inconclusive, and didn't give us the assurance that we wanted.

After receiving no reply via VHF, Steve shouted over, 'We'll go with a reference point on the boat relative to that tanker. Let's see how we go with that.'

We both agreed that the top of the navigation light on the bow was a good reference to use, and within a few minutes we could clearly see that our reference point was changing relative to the vessel, which was a good sign. I once again checked the relative bearing to the vessel, and that had clearly changed, so it was now clear to both of us that there was no risk of collision.

We were soon confident enough that it would pass by without issue, with considerable distance between us and them. Nevertheless, heart rates were certainly raised for a good few minutes, but it was a confidence-building impromptu exercise of putting our training into practice and operating as a team. It also demonstrated the necessity of always having a lookout on deck.

With calmness restored, we sat facing each other on both rowing seats. Steve was the first to break the silence.

'We deserve some rum after that.'

'Absolutely, Captain Hayes,' I replied.

After a deserved measure of rum, we both debriefed, and agreed to seek assurances from Tim and Barry that we were showing up on AIS. They were able to give us this assurance. However, we were still mystified as to why our GPS was struggling to acquire satellites and was being so temperamental.

Even after this, the boat's equipment continued to test us, not content that we'd been sufficiently terrified. We'd started the row with four fully operational autotillers, two of them brand-new. We'd named them Andy, Bill, Chris and Dave after various supporters. Two of them, Bill and Chris, were now officially deceased (the autotillers, that is, not the supporters) – cause of death: fried circuit boards, and there were worrying signs that Dave was also on his way out, as the screen display was starting to dim.

This was worrying, since we both saw this as the first sign of Dave's demise. This was causing no end of worry, since if we were left without any working autotillers, we'd need to complete the rest of the row without assisted steering, which would likely add days or even weeks on to the row. We were therefore being extra vigilant and ensuring that we were swapping the remaining two autotillers every four hours.

Doing this was a very careful operation that we did together. It would involve one of us being in the stern cabin and the other being positioned on deck. The autotiller was positioned just behind the rowing seat nearest the stern cabin. The operation was to power down, which was taken care of in the cabin. There was then a fairly swift operation of the man on deck unplugging one autotiller and quickly passing it to the man in the cabin, with a replacement autotiller handed back. This would swiftly be placed in position on the rod and plugged in, and once done we powered up again from the stern cabin. We had to do it this way to avoid excess water on any plug points and also to help avoid blown fuses. We were incredibly mindful that these were our last two autotillers, so had to take a great deal of care to not drop or clatter them on deck when passing them between us. It was like handling a newborn child.

On top of that, one of the oars snapped. On this occasion, the sea had been a tad more on the violent side than usual, and the breakage happened fairly swiftly. I'd been in the cabin asleep at the time of this incident, so on waking from my slumber and opening the cabin door, I was greeted by the sight of Steve packing away a broken oar.

The power of the ocean was something else, and, unfortunately for this oar, it had seen plenty of action since we departed La Gomera. Steve had been rowing, and the conditions had been especially lively, with some punchy and powerful waves, as well as extremely messy seas. It was just one of those things, unfortunately, and exactly the reason why we'd brought along spare oars.

'I always preferred our spare oars anyway,' mused Steve. 'They're more mature and have far more character.'

'Just like myself then, mate,' I quickly replied, despite not quite agreeing about the sentiments about the replacement oars. From memory, the handles were more coarse and incredibly sticky. The main irritation with this incident was that this oar was one of the new ones (the rest were inherited with the boat), but not to worry – we'd carried spare oars for this very reason.

Onboard entertainment had taken a hit too, and Steve's harmonica was not exactly a good substitute. Salty moisture from our enforced mini-break in the stern cabin had literally eaten into the majority of our luxury devices. All we were left with was Steve's Kindle and my iPhone. The Kindle was clearly on its way out, but my iPhone worked so long as I could continue to charge it.

Doing this was a mission in itself: I had to hold the charging cable and port up against the fan in the cabin and get everything as dry as possible before attempting to charge. I'd then need to keep wiggling the charger to find a sweet spot, which sometimes took as long as 20 minutes. Each time this occurred, it ate into my sleep time. It was a frustrating recurring exercise, but I deemed it necessary, since my phone was our only source of music, and our means for sending and receiving WhatsApp messages via the BGAN (Broadband Global Area Network, a device very much like a router that allowed us to get Wi-Fi).

This helped us, since music often helped with the more challenging shifts and took the mind off our intense bottom pain. The messages were a godsend, and we'd receive plenty from friends and family. I'd often read all of these out to Steve during our time together on deck.

Then there was the small matter of comfort. We bought several inflatable pillows and a couple of Therm-a-Rest mattresses with us – a mistake, as it turned out, as Lilly Mae wasn't exactly a smooth boat. Sharp edges and renegade bolts were in abundance, and before long we had punctures in the whole lot.

The main reason we wanted the mattresses was because they provided a great deal of comfort to the non-rower, who would sit out on deck leaning against the bow cabin while the other rowed. During the daytime, we quite liked doing this, and the non-rower would often be making water via the manual water maker or preparing daily meals, so comfort certainly helped.

We ended up resorting to using spare strips of foam, but they went missing in action after the Christmas storm. Steve then had a lightbulb moment. 'Where did you pack away those fenders, mate?' he asked. We probably had the biggest fenders on the planet, which had been deflated and packed away upon leaving La Gomera.

'Towards the back of the bow cabin. Why?'

'Grab us one and I'll reveal all,' he grinned. It was simple and obvious, but at the same time genius. I retrieved one, inflated it, and we suddenly had a squishy oversized cushion to provide some much-needed comfort – a desperate measure for desperate times!

Staying on the comfort theme, we were both spending at least 12 hours a day sitting on our sore bums, so a good seat was extremely important. During our planning phase a year out from the row, we did contemplate having them custom-made, but at £2,500 per seat, and with our sponsors' money expended, we decided that this was an investment too far, and that any unnecessary expenditure would eat into our charitable targets, which we'd set at an ambitious £50,000.

We resorted to using the seats that had served the previous owners well. These were effectively very basic sliding seats consisting of a plank of wood, layers of yoga mat foam and netting at the back to store personal effects. On balance, I think we got it right, since many things changed during the row, such as our body weight and bottoms.

To explain further, our bum bones (as I believe the medical term is) ultimately dropped through the ever-decreasing rump fat and created pressure sores where the bones pushed against the skin from the inside. The only way to help avoid this was to add extra layers of foam for comfort and then set about cutting various strategic holes in the seats. This would have been something we'd have been dismayed at doing to £2,500 seats, but with our *Blue Peter*-style seats, we were pretty relaxed about it.

Our toilet situation also took a hit. With saving space being all the rage on Lilly Mae, there wasn't room for a dedicated toilet room. All our business was done in a humble bucket, and we had three of them, which we named in the spirit of naming various things on the boat. The toilet buckets were dubbed King Richard III and Stig, while the wash bucket was named Brian. Sadly, the accumulation of days of high-protein food and the occasional curry night took its toll, culminating in Stig splitting mid-use (Steve was the culprit). Luckily, Richard III nobly stepped up to the mark and took up primary latrine duty. Brian would have been relieved to remain on wash-bucket duties for now.

Despite these shenanigans, we maintained first place in our category, even though Two-Inna-Row were gradually closing the gap. My brother Steve had been sending me daily screenshots of the leaderboard around the same time each day, and from this we were able to see our daily mileage and keep an eye on the distance between us and our nearest competitors. The updates had proved to be good motivators, but we knew our work was cut out, based on the superior boat owned by Two-Inna-Row.

In the meantime, we had our own milestones to complete. On 15 January, we finally reached the point where we had less than 1,000 miles to go – a huge morale boost, and quite a landmark. This called for rum, and double measures at that. Milestones were extremely important in this race, and we'd agreed to treat ourselves when we reached them – this certainly fit the bill.

This one in particular felt massive, since in many ways it was just under two-thirds of the race complete, and we were now into three digits, as opposed to four in terms of mileage. As usual, we downed tools for 15 minutes while jointly reflecting on the challenges and successes that had taken us to this point. I felt pretty satisfied about how we'd worked together, and with our honesty towards each other during the more challenging times.

'I reckon we're going to win mate,' I boldly declared to Steve.

There was a twinkle in his eyes as he replied, 'And I thought you weren't competitive, Petey.'

This made me chuckle, since I'd been downplaying our chances, but this was really to try to alleviate any pressure and help focus the mind on the magnitude of the challenge first and foremost. Now that we were in the thick of it, and buoyed by how we'd coped with the adversities we'd faced, I really relished the battle that lay ahead of us.

Even by this point, we were still tinkering to make things more efficient. A week or so after we got moving on 30 December, there were still times when we were finding it difficult to turn, as when the wind hit us side-on, it caught the stern cabin – a design quirk of our boat. After one particularly frustrating afternoon on 6 January, this was occurring frequently, and absolutely killing us physically as we jointly tried to bring the boat back around. We decided that enough was enough – we just couldn't face the prospect of another enforced stay in the cabin.

To combat this, we decided to remove the daggerboard. We weren't exactly in a position to change the design of the stern cabin, but figured that we'd instead focus on the hull of the boat, and no daggerboard would surely mean that it would be easier for the boat to be turned and corrected when required. It meant that the boat was more liable to tip (making an uncomfortable journey even more so, as our backsides would be sliding more), but it made it easier to row and turn the boat individually, as opposed to the joint effort and incredible stresses on our tendons. This was a real game-changer, as it allowed us both to get more rest and continue to make progress.

And rest was what we needed. We were averaging 4–5 hours of sleep a day, which may have worked for Margaret Thatcher, but she wasn't rowing across an ocean. While the boat was getting lighter as we worked through our daily food packs, we were losing a significant amount of body weight too, which wasn't exactly helping. Nothing was getting easier.

Still, there was plenty to enjoy. Night-time rowing especially was something to behold – it was cooler, and the views of the stars were incredible. There were some magical moments out there. We were often using the stars for navigational purposes, and sometimes just taking the opportunity to lay back on my rowing seat and stare up at the sky for a couple of minutes. I recall one evening row seeing a small meteor entering our atmosphere and burning up before finally disintegrating before it could hit the ocean. It was quite a cool moment, although for a moment I was concerned. Having seen too many disaster movies, I was anticipating a rather large wave coming our way, should the thing not burn up.

Plus, I seemed to find it easier to row at night. Unable to see the waves, I had to use my other senses to really 'feel' the conditions. Maybe it was psychological, but I found myself able to move with the ocean in a more efficient manner. It was for this reason that I also occasionally tried blindfold rowing during the daytime, courtesy of our manta sleeping masks.

In other good news, GPS and the chartplotter came back to life for a few days. We were so used to it not working that we were happy enough for our stand-in system of navigating via manual compass and getting regular feedback via satellite phone text message from our weather router, Tim. However, on the rare occasions that it did come back to life, we could obviously get more clarity on our exact position and course overground. It would also make our two-hour rowing shifts far more interesting, since we'd compete with each other in a fun way, and see how many nautical miles we could clock in each stint.

Steve also managed to find my hair clippers during a routine sort-out in the cabin.

'Why have you brought these along, mate?' were his words, to which I replied, 'I didn't want to be looking like a circus clown on arrival in Antigua.'

This would be on account of being folically challenged and my hair perhaps not growing back on the top as quickly as the sides, so I'd fully intended to go grade one all over, but keep the beard. Steve soon put a halt to these proceedings by asking Barry to put out a poll and let the public decide. The result was a fairly unanimous 'no trim' decision, so the clippers were redundant – that is, apart from one use, which will be disclosed in Chapter 15, just before arrival into Antigua. Sorry voters.

We continued to go with the winds and conditions, averaging a very healthy 65 miles per day over a couple of weeks while not fighting the conditions too much. We'd also adjusted nicely to the feel of the boat minus the daggerboard. The only drawback here was that the redundant daggerboard was now a guest in our stern cabin, giving us less room to stretch out. These first two weeks of January would prove to be our best in terms of daily mileage for the entire row. We were still getting bashed around on frequent occasions, but a few bruises were a fair exchange for decent progress.

Interlude 11

WITH THE bad weather mostly behind us, we were able to escape the sweat box and get on with the task of rowing across the Atlantic. We returned to our routine and tried to enjoy the experience as much as possible. My phone had died a while back, which removed a large amount of my freedom and independence. Pete would let me use his phone to check WhatsApp and read messages, etc., but they were mostly messages for him, and I didn't want to use the phone if he wasn't, and didn't want to be responsible if our last bit of tech died.

Thankfully, I was able to call my wife daily, but even the satellite phones were starting to become very temperamental, as anything with a charging port starts to corrode from the sea water/sea air.

Social media became a large discussion point for each day, and one of our priorities was to get as much content back to Barry, our social media manager, as possible. Our row had come soon after the Covid lockdowns, so not a lot of positive stuff had happened in Jersey for a while (there was a fatal gas explosion a couple of days after we'd arrived in La Gomera, as well as a boat sinking), so we were always very keen to provide a good news story and something for the residents of our little island to get behind. We'd also paid him to post several posts per day across different platforms, so it would have been a waste of money if we didn't get anything back to him!

Once the first few weeks were out of the way, life at sea became quite mundane. Not in a bad way; more in a simplistic way. There was always something to fix, and always something to look at, whether that be the shape of the waves, the shape of the clouds, the sunrises, the sunsets, the starry nights ... but without pictures it all became a rather mundane story for Barry to translate to our families and followers back home.

Having invested in some fishing gear, I daydreamed about catching a marlin. These magnificent fish had caused quite a lot of drama in the ocean-rowing community in the past few years, spearing several boats and causing a lot of worry. As I sat rowing, half asleep, sometimes with my eyes closed and sleep mask on, I'd have childish dreams of wrestling a marlin into the boat and holding it up, just for the photos to send back to Barry. I'd also daydreamed about cleaning the underside of the boat and being approached by a shark, only to stab it like Leonardo DiCaprio in *The Beach*, and become the hero of the fleet. Sleep deprivation and monotony clearly do weird things to the mind.

Thankfully, Sundays became something to look forward to. To anyone that knows Pete and me, it will come as no surprise to learn that we're both partial to a wee tipple on occasion. To be honest, most of our time spent together is usually under the influence of alcohol. A meet-up to discuss the row website = two bottles of red. A family gathering at Christmas = many bottles of everything. Two weeks in La Gomera = 296 pints of lager and a lost pair of shoes!

Out here, we had limited rations: two litres of Havana Club 7 rum, two quarter-bottles of red wine, and I think a couple of quarter-bottles of sparkling wine. The wine was finished over the Christmas period, but the rum was rationed out by me, not Pete the accountant – 2000ml rum divided by two rowers, one of which doesn't like spirits much, divided by an anticipated finish time of about 50 days/seven weeks = about 150ml rum per person per week. Roughly.

Anyway, every Sunday evening at around 8pm (sunset), we'd take a break from rowing for 10–20 minutes and enjoy some rum while reflecting on the previous week, chatting about anything and discussing what we were most looking forward to when we reached Antigua. On reflection, I think that was the most beneficial thing we could have done during our row, and I'd strongly encourage every team to do something similar – time out to do a little SWOT analysis, stroke each other's egos and focus on the future.

Obviously, one of us would have to carry on rowing while tipsy, and the other could go and sleep off their six (normal UK) measures of rum for two hours before having to groggily jump on the oars. I suppose it's okay to admit now that Pete never got much rum, and I always filled my cup/glass/receptacle more, but I think he knew that.

Steve Hayes

Chapter 12

California dreamin'

EVER SINCE I started ultrarunning, completing the Western States 100 had been an ambition of mine. Established in 1977, it has the distinction of being the oldest ultra in the United States. Starting at Squaw Valley (since renamed Olympic Valley), California, and traversing the historic Western States trail, runners ascend 18,000ft and descend nearly 23,000ft before they reach the finish line at Placer High School in Auburn, California. As such, a place on the starting line is incredibly sought-after.

The thing is, not just anyone can claim entry; you have to be entered into a lottery, which you can only become eligible for by completing a qualifying event, which is generally another 100-mile ultramarathon. In this case, mine happened to be the Lakeland 100 in 2015.

My genesis with the Western States started sometime in 2016 when I sat down and commenced what I thought would be a long-term plan for gaining entry to this race. Since this was the first time I'd tried to enter, I was aware that I'd only be allocated one lottery ticket. This meant that I effectively had next to no chance, as the idea is that each year thereafter, your lottery allocation doubles, so you have a greater chance as the years progress, assuming you keep on trying. Once my entry had been submitted, I mentally switched off and began to think about what races would be more realistic for 2017.

Yet, life has a habit of surprising you. Fast-forward to December 2016, I'd just completed the Dorset Half-Marathon with Andy McDonald. We were enjoying a few frothy ales in a pub in Wareham when my friend from back home, Leanne Rive, texted me with a message that read, 'Oh my God, Congratulations.'

On replying to her and explaining that my time hadn't exactly been that spectacular, I realised that she meant something else. After checking my emails, I worked out what she meant: I'd been pulled from the hat for the Western States 2017. What immediately followed was a call to Rachel, starting, 'Well, you'll never guess what …'

Shock didn't cover it. Reality soon set in, though – this was really happening. And I was up against it. The cut-off time for finishing is 30 hours – a tough enough challenge without taking into account the fact that this would involve a lot of moving fairly swiftly in the heat and humidity, which definitely wasn't my forte.

I was already training for another ultra, so fitness wasn't an issue. Ever the pragmatist, I studied the race's profile and drafted a rough pacing plan that estimated a finish time of 27 hours.

My studies produced another dilemma, however, this time concerning logistics. Since the race start and finish were in very different locations, and I also had to factor in my incoming and outgoing flights, I sent an email to the race director with a general query around this. He advised me to get myself set up with a support crew, pointing to an area on the website where I could find one.

The prospect of a support crew was somewhat alien to me, since I was very used to being self-sufficient and generally fending for myself. My initial thought was that a support crew fussing over me would make things more complicated, but I was willing to open myself up to a new experience, and it seemed to be how it was done at the Western States.

Finding one proved to be a bit like a matchmaking concept, where runners and potential crew put their details out there, leaving it down to you to make contact. As luck would have it, I got in touch with a chap called Michael Li from San Francisco, and we had a good chat over Skype. We hit it off, and I knew I was in good hands. Mike was keen to hear about my background, so I started listing everything I'd done since the MDS in 2013. Reading it back, it dawned on me: I was starting to build up a bit of a race CV.

'Those races are great, but you're soon to experience the best race in the world.' Mike's words perfectly melded ringing endorsement with the promise of the adventure of a lifetime.

Mike was amazing right from the start of the process, and was the font of knowledge for anything to do with the race, having crewed for a couple of runners in previous years. He arranged to meet me on arrival into San Francisco, and spent the following day giving me a guided tour of the city – as an afterthought, we even fitted in a couple of runs! One of them turned out to be a very scenic ten-miler going over the Golden Gate Bridge, hitting a few trails on the other side and then back over the bridge. Mike then drove the both of us to Squaw Valley ahead of the race. The rough plan was that he'd crew me, and perhaps run the final 20 miles with me.

While I was happy with my pre-race preparation, it was a different story when I arrived in San Francisco on the Tuesday before, ready for the drive to Squaw Valley. I kept waking up at around 3am, which wasn't exactly a good thing, since I was steadily becoming more and more sleep deprived, only averaging about five hours of sleep in the four or so nights leading up to race day. I really don't know why this was – I can only put it down to nerves.

On the flight out, I was really feeling the pressure. This race felt like a one-time chance on account of it being so difficult to secure entry. I desperately wanted to do myself justice out there, and could only imagine my grumpiness on the return flight home should I DNF. I was dealing with tight cut-offs as well as significant heat and humidity, and the race statistics did suggest that a DNF was a strong possibility.

I also ended up with a splitting headache the night before – another impediment to getting any sleep. The race was to start in the very early hours, so, with my head imploding, I succumbed to a strong painkiller, which only just managed to squash it and get me an hour's sleep before I needed to be up again. Having one last WhatsApp call with Rachel just before I left the hotel room for the race, I got a glimpse of my panic-stricken face on WhatsApp just before the call connected, which was pretty funny in hindsight, but not so much at the time.

Mike was there to meet me at the start and provide me with some motivational words: 'You're ready, dude. Now's your time. Seize the day!'

I was buzzing as I stood shoulder to shoulder with the other competitors of this prestigious race. The combined sound of numerous excitable conversations were ringing in my ears, and the bright lights of smartphones were everywhere, recording every moment.

Meanwhile, Mike took up position to record the race start and had even brought a ladder along so he could get a clear view of the race start. I saw him take up his position and shout to the crowds, 'Get your cowbells ready, folks. Western States baby, whoo hoo!'

I was now eagerly awaiting the countdown, while having a good catch-up with fellow UK competitor, Tremayne Cowdry, who I'd met on some previous races. Tremayne is a very good runner and always has a smile on his face, and it was really good to catch up with him. It certainly helped ease my nerves a little.

The countdown arrived, with everyone calling ten down to one, and then we were off to the sound of a shotgun blast (Western States tradition), mass whooping and the clatter of cowbells. Mike was easy to spot on his ladder as I ran past.

'Alright Pete. Go get 'em,' followed quickly by, '100 miles in one day, baby!' It remains the most incredible race start I've ever been a part of.

I knew there was a solid 2,400ft of ascent awaiting me, but this was over good trail. I pushed forwards, alternating a steady power-walk with a light jog on the ups while running the flats. It was interesting to observe the different-sized packs and attire of the competitors. Some were shirtless, carrying a couple of handhelds with belts, while others were fully kitted with ten-litre packs.

The initial climb was comfortable, and I was pleased with how I'd started. However, as I expected, we hit snow at 1,800ft, which remained for the rest of the ascent. This was going to be a long day after all.

Before long, I reached Watson's Monument (named for Robert Watson, a legendary explorer who helped mark the trail), where we'd begin our first descent. The trainers I'd chosen (New Balance Leadvilles) were decent enough on trails, but I was slipping quite a lot on the snow. Mindful of sustaining an early injury, I leaned forward, basically trying to foot-ski the slope, but occasionally it was easier to control the descent by simply using my nice, padded backside and sliding down. Crampons and poles weren't permitted, and both would have come in handy at this point. What this approach lacked in style, it made up for by reducing the risk of catching an ankle or twisting a limb.

Eventually, the snow gave way to trail and mud, which introduced a new dilemma. I noticed many competitors making great efforts to dance around the puddles. I knew there was no long-term way to avoiding a foot-soaking, so I just ran through the middle. My Leadvilles would flush out easily enough, and my feet were always going to hurt, so I figured that I'd deal with that later on. Sock changes would be an option, too.

After the checkpoint at Red Star Ridge, there was significantly less mud and snow, leaving a decent trail to follow. It was long, under a canopy of trees and full of switchbacks, made much more challenging by the rapidly increasing temperatures and humidity. It was now 9am, and I'd been taking salt tablets on the hour and keeping a steady fluid intake. However, I was sweating a great deal and already feeling hamstring stiffness and cramping. Also, my fluid intake since the previous checkpoint had been exceptionally high, and I knew I was going to run out of water before Duncan Canyon, so I had to ration myself for the final hour before the checkpoint.

I'd given Mike a target time for Duncan Canyon of 10.20am, and early on I really felt that I was going to exceed this target. However, the snow and mud took its toll, and I ended up coming into Duncan Canyon – and the 23-mile mark – over an hour after my planned time: 11.30am, worryingly close to cut-off. I couldn't reconcile this in my head, since I knew there were so many competitors behind me. The reason for the high DNF rate was starting to become very clear.

On entering Duncan Canyon, I must have looked a mess. The game plan was certainly not to feel like shit with 77 miles to go. As I ran in, I could see Mike frantically waving his arms.

'Pete! Pete!' he shouted. 'Give me your bottles!' Like myself, he must have been slightly nervous about my later-than-planned arrival. Nevertheless, he was first-class, and managed the transition as planned. It felt like a F1 pit stop as he shoved an ice-packed buff around my neck, filled my cooling sleeves with ice and refilled my soft flasks. He also gave me a sandwich bag full of frozen fruit, which looked perfect, before kicking my sorry arse out of the checkpoint.

I felt very deflated because of how close I was to cut-off. However, I wasn't going to let Mike down, given all the time and effort he'd put into planning his crew duties, so I refocused on getting moving. The ice got to work quickly, and I found myself picking up a very good pace, which in turn started to reduce my stress levels.

Unfortunately, and somewhat inevitably, I then started cramping in both hamstrings. I stopped and made efforts to sort that out while also trying to get my core temperature down. I took the opportunity to have a quick look at my target times. This turned out to be an inspired move – after the next checkpoint, the race profile looked easier, and could present me with an opportunity to settle down and pick up my pace. My game plan was to get into Robinson Flat with my body in check, then focus on making up time.

Mike's neck-buff idea was feeling more inspired by the second. He called this his secret weapon, and the neck-buff pocket allowed for ice to be stored towards the back for regular top-ups, which really helped with keeping my body temperature down. I topped up my running sleeves with ice to do the same.

I'd lost the stiffness and cramps, and was adopting a well-used tactic of running in the shade while occasionally walking in the sun. I entered Robinson Flat and the Miller's Defeat aid station (named for being the site of a historic mining dispute) feeling good, buoyed by the fact that I was now moving further ahead of the cut-offs. Positivity breeds positivity, and all of this was helping my morale.

Also, the crew were providing me with insights, telling me that the course was as good as it got for the next few miles ahead, so I knew this was a golden opportunity to make these miles count. With 100-milers, banking time ahead of cut-offs while you can is key, since you always have to expect the unexpected at some point, and your time buffer can help to deal with this.

After what felt like some respectable miles, I reached Dusty Corners feeling in good shape. I think Mike could see the difference, and it was encouraging that I'd put myself in a much better place.

Here, I met Ed Liu and Ken Reicher for the first time. Good friends with Mike, they were very familiar with the Western States route. They also were very generous to the running community, and certainly took me under their wing that day, meticulously preparing for any fuel or hydration need I may require. Ken offered me a deckchair, but I politely declined on account of knowing how much of a challenge it would be to get back up again.

They were both offering amazing words of encouragement, which helped maintain my good spirits. The whole crew were explaining what was coming up next, which involved another descent into a canyon, followed by an almighty climb back up.

Mike said, 'When you reach the waterfall, take five minutes and get in.'

Ken concurred: 'Every time you see a stream, dunk yourself in.' It was all good advice, and would help me to regulate my body temperature. Already, they felt like lifelong friends. That's the ultrarunning community for you.

I felt very proud of myself for the comeback and for not letting the predicament get in my head too much at Duncan Canyon. Mike had the checkpoint system nailed. He's very methodical and organised, and knew exactly what I needed. I ran out of there feeling upbeat, knowing that I had kind terrain ahead to Last Chance, and the opportunity to make up some more time.

I ran out of the checkpoint en route to Devil's Thumb feeling very confident. All that stood between me and mile 48 was a 2,000ft descent into the canyon, followed by a rather steep 2,000ft climb back out again.

The descent was very energy-sapping in the rising heat and humidity, with constant switchbacks – it just went on and on. We were also under a canopy of trees, which added humidity to the already 'bloody hot' equation. This, I found, was very similar to the conditions I'd dealt with on the Jungle Marathon. Anticipating this, I'd taken a little treat from Last Chance (a banana). What really kept me going was the thought of a nice dip in the creek, followed by an injection of banana energy, before attempting the climb back up.

I was well-trained on the climbs, so kept a steady striding rhythm, but it was tough. I passed many people doubled over, some being sick. I could understand this, since I was starting to feel light-headed myself. I offered support, but was always given the thumbs-up. I guess everyone has their way of dealing with the climbs but, nevertheless, I wanted to check on the wellbeing of anyone I passed.

After what felt like ages of being slowly roasted alive, I reached Devil's Thumb. I felt very dizzy on reaching the top, which was unsurprising, given the conditions. Upon arriving, we were each provided with an ice lolly, which – the biggest setback of the day – I promptly dropped in the dirt. However, a dirt-flavoured lolly was not something to pass up, and would surely have additional nutrients, so I polished that off without fuss, hoping the bugs within would contain some slow-release energy for the next section.

The next part involved a long descent into El Dorado Creek. This was more gradual, but seemed even more endless, taking us 2,600ft down. I felt fresh enough in my legs and good on my feet, but was mindful of keeping my core body temperature in check, as well as taking my salts and electrolytes. Even so, the creek didn't appear to be getting any closer. I tried to switch off and just visualise lying in it. This kept my limbs moving closer to the goal.

Upon reaching the checkpoint at El Dorado Creek, I headed straight for the water and submerged. I just laid on my back, staring up at the sky, and took a moment to listen to the sounds around me. It was a beautiful moment, and provided me with the energy and state of mind to tackle the ascent.

Upon leaving, one of the checkpoint crew told me that this climb, even though 1,800ft high, wasn't as steep, and that there would actually be runnable parts. I left with my customary bag of fruit and began my power-walk onwards to Michigan Bluff. This was to be mile 56, and would provide my third opportunity to catch up with Mike.

Running into Michigan Bluff was just electric. There was a large crowd, and the cheers were a huge lift. They were giving a big shout-out to each runner as they came in, so it was good to hear my announcement: '… from the island of Jersey!'

There was still 44 miles to go, but in my mind I'd dealt with the early snow and then the heat. I was well hydrated and time was on my side. The legs were feeling significantly more worked than at Last Chance – an early sign that the back-to-back creeks had taken their toll.

As usual, Mike got to work rummaging in the supplies box and starting to get all my soft flasks topped up. Meanwhile, I was pacing around, grabbing any food that looked slightly appealing – generally cold fruit.

Various people were saying, 'Runner, you're looking good.' I was feeling a little beaten-up physically, but very positive mentally, and the well-wishes were boosting this. Mike sorted the ice buff, handed me another sandwich bag full of cold fruit pieces, and we started to leave the checkpoint to the sound of cheers and cowbells.

Mike told me that he'd been keeping Rachel updated on Facebook, and what to expect next. 'Six miles to Foresthill: three up, two down and one flat. After Foresthill, it's mostly downhill.'

I knew it was around six miles to Foresthill, and the profile Mike explained helped. Mike made me chuckle when I explained that various parts of the course had been a killer so far. He replied, 'Walmsley dropped. You're better than that Walmsley dude.'

Jim Walmsley had been the race favourite, so hearing this was a big shock (he has since gone on to win the race four times, including setting a course record in 2018, before bettering his own time the following year, so it's probably fair to say that he got over it!).

I thought I'd be able to hammer out the six miles before it got dark. The way I was feeling, I could see this taking a little over an hour, so I told Mike I'd grab my head torch at Foresthill and see him there shortly. I also handed him back the head torch I had on me, since that was fairly low on battery from the race start. That was a mistake on my behalf, since I was heading into forest for this six-mile stretch.

I left Michigan Bluff running, and did so for the next mile or so. However, I was entering a forest, and it was now very evident that it would be dark long before I reached the next checkpoint. One fellow runner and his pacer allowed me to run between them and share their light, for which I was hugely grateful. I'd sat with this guy in two of the creeks, and was later very pleased to see he completed this race. This tactic worked really well until a pacer friend of Mike's, Kirsten, lent me a hand torch, which enabled me to move forwards independently.

Strangely, working with torchlight marked an unexpected – and negative – turning point. The physical exertions of the last 15 hours had taken their toll, as well as the lack of sleep in the run-up to the event. As soon as darkness descended, I became very tired. I slowed down to an ungainly shuffle coming into Foresthill. In the space of four miles I'd transformed from a man with a spring in his step to a lumbering, very old wildebeest.

I debated over what to change at Foresthill after I met with Mike. We stood at the back of his car, and all I wanted to do was clamber in and get some sleep. However, I was very conscious that I was only one hour and 45 minutes ahead of cut-off, so I put that thought out of my head as quickly as I could.

My feet were now very sore and wet – each step felt like walking on broken glass. However, I saw little value in foot care at this point, and just figured the feet would continue to get wet and there would be suffering involved for these experienced trotters, so I'd have to resort to painkillers eventually. I'd dealt with these scenarios before, so I knew I could get through it. The only thing I changed was to put a clean running top on. In hindsight, I should have kept the other one on, since the smell was actually keeping me awake.

Mike could see the state I was in.

'Tell you what,' he said, 'I'll run with you out of Foresthill.'

I replied, 'I don't think there will be a whole lot of running due to my feet, but I'd love the company mate, and I'll be doing my best to get going again. The painkillers should kick in soon enough.'

While his assistance was welcome, it didn't change the facts of my physical condition. I was stumbling and tripping at every opportunity. Mike was keeping a close eye on me. I was very tired, and really struggling with communication from my brain to my feet. Mike could see that I was in trouble, and encouraged me to slow right down and follow his lead with a steady hike.

'Take your time. It's cooler, but you're in the dark descending a lot. I don't want you to trip.'

He followed up with, 'I'll get you down to the bottom of the first descent, and then turn back.'

He was also busy talking on his mobile, making arrangements – I was dreading the point where he'd head back to Foresthill. Our pre-race plan was for him to pace me from mile 80, so I knew he'd need to double back soon to retrieve the car and meet me later on.

To my surprise, he didn't turn back, staying with me all the way to CAL1. Then, he surprised me again with some more news. 'I've sorted out the logistics,' he said. 'Looks like I'll be seeing you in all the way to the finish!'

I was absolutely ecstatic, even though it would have been hard to discern from my tired, baggy face. It was a typically selfless gesture from a guy who had already pulled out all the stops to ensure I'd finish this race, and have a good time while doing so. He'd been awake just as long as me, and been working like an absolute trooper at all the checkpoints. It was an incredible gesture.

We slowly power-hiked through the night to Rucky Chucky. CAL2 and CAL3 came and went – it was a slow, dark blur. I was deeply frustrated that I couldn't pick up the pace, since the terrain and profile were actually pretty decent. Even though it was dark, it felt very muggy, and I couldn't shake off the tiredness. The best tactic was to try to maintain 15-minute miles. To attempt anything else would have no doubt resulted in a fall or an ankle twist. I'd read many blogs about this race, and each contained a chapter where the wheels well and truly fell off. Well, I was now living out my own version.

The night was slow, but we eventually reached Rucky Chucky. By now, I was trying to run, but each step still felt like running on broken glass. However, sore feet and tiredness were not going to be a reason for a DNF. I still had some good time in the bank, and was ahead of cut-offs.

Strangely, I thought back to an unintended motivational line that Steve Hayes had spoken to me in a race called 'Escape from Meriden' the previous year. His exact words were: 'Stop being a pussy.' At the time it wasn't what I wanted to hear, so I was absolutely raging at him. However, on this occasion, I resolved to follow his advice. I also reflected once again on the low odds of me even doing this race, and reminded myself how lucky I was to be here.

Rucky Chucky was a quick checkpoint, and within five minutes of arrival we were being rowed across the river so we could pick up the trail again. Getting in and out of the boat with lead-weight legs was a comedy affair, but it was nice to take the load off in the boat just for a minute or so.

Upon reaching the other side, we were faced with a 25–30-minute climb to Green Gate. It was a steady climb over good terrain, and I was about to reach mile 80. I was still very much in control, and looking forward to sunrise and what I hoped would bring a new lease of life. This was normally the case, based on my experience in races to date.

At Green Gate, I once again started thinking tactically. The next 10–11 miles looked like a good opportunity to pick up the pace. My feet were in a bad way, but I needed to get them used to running again. Mike took the lead, and we'd continue on a steady, fast hike and run where possible.

The first section to Auburn Lake Trails was more difficult, with a few climbs, while the section to Quarry Road was more kind. Small climbs were starting to feel mountainous on tired limbs and sore feet. However, around 5.30am, daylight arrived, allowing me to turn the head torch off. I found that the fog of tiredness that had been clinging to me was disappearing, and running was becoming more frequent. I dread to think what I actually looked like, but it felt good to be moving relatively quickly again.

The run to Quarry Road was the fastest I'd moved since mile 60. Mike was expertly dictating the pace, and keeping the pressure on to run as much as possible.

'Just follow my lead, dude. Two minutes run, and then two minutes walk.' He knew I was in pain, but you're always going to be when you're 91 miles into a 100-mile race! However, he recognised when to get me running and when to slow down. This guy was truly my guardian angel. It was at this point that I took my first and only painkiller, since the feet were starting to hit a new level in the pain locker.

Reaching Quarry Road was monumental for me. It was 7.20am, and I had three hours and 40 minutes to carve out just over nine miles. Marking this occasion, I had a celebratory toilet stop, a private wobbly-lip moment, and saddled up for the next stint.

The next 3.5 miles to Pointed Rocks was as tough as expected, given that it was mostly ascending and the

California heat was rising fast. The pace was not quick, but fast enough to keep me on for a sub-30-hour finish. I reflected that I'd managed the race well – I'd put myself in a position where I could finish this at walking pace if I wanted to. However, it was a running race, and I was still determined to do as much of this as I possibly could. This had been a particularly tough year, underlined by the completion rate being 67.2 per cent. Ordinarily, it would have been around 80 per cent. This higher than usual rate of dropouts can be put down to the unusually inhospitable conditions: heavy snow at the start making it slow going initially, followed by very high temperatures for the rest of the event.

I had a quick chat with Mike about the route, and what was left.

'It's all downhill to No Hands Bridge,' he said. Therefore, I took the time to cool down for a good penultimate section. Sure enough, Mike and I moved swiftly through to No Hands. On entering, a fellow competitor looked like he was in big trouble, struggling to stay on his feet. Nonetheless, he waved away any support – his exact words were, 'Fuck off! Fuck off!'

He could be forgiven for the strong language – you're effectively disqualified if you're physically aided or supported during the race. Fortunately, I had no such drama at No Hands, and jogged across, chatting to Mike.

'It's 9.10 right now,' he said. 'If we can get to Robie Point by 10am, we've got an hour to clear that final mile. We can walk it!'

I asked how far it was to Robie Point from here, and he replied, 'Two miles, and you've got 50 minutes to do it. Easy!'

A satisfied smile spread across my face. I had one hour and 50 minutes to complete three miles, then I'd completed the race. Bloody hell!

On the drive up to Squaw Valley on the Thursday, Mike had taken me to both the finish line and mile 99 so that I could visualise everything. This was a good tactic, as I could picture that sign at mile 99. I was looking forward to reaching it, knowing that it was a mile of simple tarmac downhill from there.

The climb to Robie Point was fine by me, since I knew it was the last climb of a day. Psychologically, I could find those hidden energy reserves somewhere within.

The cheers at Robie Point were something else, resulting in a second wobbly-lip moment. I reflect on many things before the end of races, and this had truly been an epic. I'd literally given everything both physically and mentally. What had made this event more special was the support and encouragement I'd received throughout, and from Mike in particular. I truly hope I can repay the favour one day.

Mike had been posting Facebook updates and videos throughout the day, and had allowed my family and close friends to be part of the race with me. I knew throughout that he was doing this, and it really did help. Sure enough, I had my picture taken at the mile 99 sign, and then began my descent to Placer High School.

Mike recorded the final mile, and it was a rollercoaster of cheers, high-fives and general goodwill. I was offered a beer, which I apologetically refused, but Mike collected it on my behalf, and ultimately looked after it until the finish. Again, top bloke.

I wanted to run all of the final mile, but had to walk occasionally to compose myself and allow the incredible pain in my feet to ease off. About 500m from the finish, Craig Thornley, the race director, with an amazing nine finishes under his belt, ran past me. This seemed like a good point to slow down, walk and get myself in the zone.

After a minute, I began the run to the athletics track. Entering the stadium was spine-tingling. Mike was continuing to record my every move, screaming encouragement. As I started to hear the noise erupt from the stadium, Mike shouted, 'Listen to this! Come on! This is all for you!' I felt like I was in dreamland, and the energy from the stadium carried me around the track.

Mike encouraged me to move to the middle lane (for the cameras), and his final emotional words to me before I crossed the line were, 'I'm so fucking proud of you, dude.' With those words ringing in my ears, I crossed the line with arms held aloft at 29:13.

My first thought was to seek out the guy who had put so much into my race and had acted as the best support and friend for the entire journey. Mike and I had done it, and I was bloody ecstatic.

Post-race, I reflect on the Western States as one of the best endurance experiences of my life. It receives many plaudits, and rightly so. The event is magical, made more so by the never-ending support, kindness and friendship offered throughout by all involved.

This was a high point for me in so many respects – which was just as well, as things were about to take a downward turn on several levels.

Interlude 12.1

AS FAR back as I can remember, my father has always been doing insane challenges, such as ultramarathons through the Sahara desert, the Arctic Circle and the Amazon rainforest, to name a few. I didn't think there was anything different about it at the time. Didn't everyone's dads do stuff like this for fun?

Despite this, I thought that the Atlantic row was too crazy, even for him. My initial reaction was that of disbelief due to the incredible difficulty that the race posed. However, I still believed he could do it.

The toughest part for me was the start as I saw him go past the horizon, knowing that it could be as much as three months before I saw him again. This included my 16th birthday, which was pretty tough. However, I still managed to contact him via daily messages and video calls.

Throughout the months following, I managed to track his progress through the app – I let him know how he was getting on, which I hoped provided some motivation!

While I was proud of him, I did fear for him at a number of points. The unforgiving seas were a terrifying thought, so the videos of the 30ft waves surrounding him that he sent to us didn't help! He thought they were no big deal, and just carried on rowing.

His race wasn't all terror and fear; he managed to send a lot of cheery videos throughout the race, including the stunning views and encounters with sea life such as dolphins. I also received a concerning number of videos of his rowing partner, Steve, and his lack of clothes.

The time away paid off as it was great to see him when he finally returned home, more shrivelled and hairier than before. The time spent away was definitely hard, but was worth it for him to accomplish such a milestone.

I've recently been more involved in running and keeping up my fitness, and he has been there to help me throughout my journey, which I'm grateful for. Despite being 52, he's still speeding past me in most runs. I aim to surpass him one day!

Josh Wright, Pete's son

Interlude 12.2

MY DAD is truly one of the most amazing people I've met. He has taught me how to be a kind and respectful person, to have self-confidence, and that it doesn't matter if you're not the best at something; trying is more important.

I first remember him doing fundraisers and charity work when I was about five. I was in the kitchen with Mum, and she was showing me photos of my dad in the jungle, trekking through murky lakes and sleeping in hammocks. I was amazed. I told my whole class and all my teachers and everyone that my dad was in the jungle. Everyone was impressed, but not as much as I was.

From when I was little, I mainly remember small snippets of him treating me like a princess and being carried around wherever I was. One of these was when he was training for the car pull. I had to sit on this big tyre and be pulled around for hours every week. I didn't mind it – to be honest, I enjoyed it. He seemed very strong compared to every other dad.

I remember finding out my dad was rowing the Atlantic, and I wasn't too thrilled, to be honest, when I found out. I didn't want him to get swallowed by a megalodon or something. But still, I was proud and happy for my dad, and wanted him to do what he wanted with his life if it made him happy.

Over the two months he was gone, I really missed him.

I'm very lucky to have a dad like mine; he's adventurous, wild, strong. But mainly he's kind, caring and soft-hearted. The reason he does these marathons is to raise money for people who need it more than him and to make memories along the way. I love my dad.

Leila Wright, Pete's daughter

Chapter 13

Getting closer

IT'S IMPOSSIBLE to overstate how big a psychological impact knowing that we had less than 1,000 miles to go was.

'We've done the hard bit, mate. The rest will be a doddle,' I joked to Steve.

'The pioneers of old would be paying homage to us if they could see us in full flow now,' replied Steve.

We were never shy to congratulate ourselves, but we were equally mindful that the sea can be a cruel mistress, and that anything can happen at any time, whether it be one nautical mile or 1,000. With that in mind, we resolved to keep doing what we were doing: have lots of fun, and stay respectful of the unpredictable environment we were inhabiting.

Buoyed by hitting this landmark, we immediately started planning ahead. I'd sit on my comfortable fender cushion with my back against the bow cabin while Steve rowed, doing the maths and basing it on our current mileage up to mid-January. From this, I picked out 31 January as a realistic arrival date into Antigua. We'd been making very good progress, establishing a solid routine of two hours on and two hours off. Naturally, we felt that we were becoming more experienced as we went along. It therefore seemed very logical to be optimistic.

As it turned out, this was a big mistake.

Almost the moment we dropped down to triple digits, the conditions started to conspire against us. The wind slowed right down, as did any other assist from the underlying currents. The lack of weather is far more of a problem than it sounds: shorn of the natural elements' propensity to propel us along, we slowed right down.

Couple this with the blisteringly hot sunshine (the clouds had taken a leave of absence, too), and we were starting to really feel every stroke of the oar. The gains slowed right down, as did our daily mileage.

Confidence-wise, this was a big blow. The possibility of making it to the finish line by the end of January started to evaporate, and this really started to impact us. Up until our purple patch of great daily mileage in the first half of January, we hadn't really been thinking ahead to exactly when we'd finish, taking each day as it came. Since we were spurred on by the thought of breaking through the 1,000-miles-to-go barrier, we started to allow ourselves to anticipate finishing and set ourselves daily targets in terms of feasible mileage. The conditions slowing down made these targets unattainable, and our morale took a big hit as we saw our estimated time of arrival inexorably pushed back.

What also took a hit was our respective bodies from unwanted ocean visitors: flying fish. These creatures would leap from the sea, transferring from water to air as if there were no boundaries, and then smoothly glide along, changing direction mid-flight, and remaining airborne for up to 45 seconds at a time. Unfortunately, in the dark of night, these fish didn't seem to be able to see where they were going, resulting in a fair number of them meeting an early demise as they either trapped themselves or smashed into our boat. Or us.

Their kamikaze somersaults became an increasingly frequent occurrence. Disposing of their decomposing bodies was added to the 'essential chores' list, as they'd end up all over deck, seemingly in every nook and cranny. Their stench was not pleasant either, necessitating their quick removal, often at the expense of valuable rowing time.

This unwanted aqua assault culminated on one of my night shifts, where I already wasn't having the best of times. Having just been utterly drenched by a heavy, squally shower, I was now cold and feeling even more sleep deprived than I'd become used to. I'd also had trouble charging my phone due to moisture detection, so was taking on this shift without any music – a tough prospect, facing the ocean without the *Rocky* or *Top Gun* soundtrack.

Having sat down to row, I commenced what had now become automatic. Then, out of nowhere, I received an almighty slap to the right-hand side of my face. Reeling, I looked down to see a flying fish flapping in the footwell. I was absolutely raging, and quickly picked the thing up and threw it back into the ocean. There's nothing quite like receiving a great big slap when you're having a tough day.

Steve had his turn five days later – it took him from behind and smacked into his back, after which it was unceremoniously dumped back to where it came from. Steve said he spat on it first, and called it the 'c' word before returning it to the ocean. My fish got off lightly, it seems.

With our daily mileage slowing down, and our physical efforts doubling in the increasingly hot conditions, we were still manually pumping water in between our two-hour rowing shifts. It's fair to say that we were running on empty, and even began to explore the possibility of whether we'd be able to start drinking our ballast water. Ours was one of the only boats in the fleet that was required, based on its design, to have around 100 litres of ballast water stored. This added weight – roughly 100kg – to what was already a very heavy boat.

The purpose behind the ballast water would be to enable the boat to self-right in the event of capsizing. We therefore knew that if we were to be allowed to drink any of the fresh ballast water stored, we'd need to immediately refill it with salt water and store it back so that the integrity of the boat wasn't compromised. While this meant that we'd receive no advantage by reducing the weight of the boat's contents, we at least might be able to take a break from manually pumping water and get ourselves properly hydrated, and perhaps some more sleep over and above our current four hours per day. We therefore began to explore this option with Atlantic Campaigns.

Also, Two-Inna-Row were continuing to catch up with us – something we were uncomfortably aware of, being able to track their progress on a daily basis courtesy of daily updates from my brother. We were now rowing west and effectively cutting through the wind that was blowing from the north. This made it slow going for us, as well as very heavy at the oars. Ultimately, we'd need to get further south at some point, but we also didn't want to drop south too early and risk being more south than Antigua on our anticipated approach.

Worst case, this could leave us with an almighty late battle to make it to Antigua, and also risk being swept past the island, so we wanted to keep this advantage in our back pocket for now. We were keeping an eye on our daily mileage, compared to Two-Inna-Row, and could see they were gaining on us each day by two to three miles. It felt like it was a matter of time before they took first place from us.

In day-to-day rowing, as we battled to keep hold of our lead, it almost became a case of waiting for things to go wrong – and indeed, there were plenty of things that could: rudder, autotiller, oars, GPS and navigation, personal injury, inability to make water. There were so many things that could break down and delay us. We lived in a constant state of anxiety about the number of things that were outside of our control. We were not left disappointed.

On 18 January, in the middle of the night, as I was attempting one of my sleeping shifts, I received the dreaded knock on the cabin door far earlier than it was due. That meant that there was a problem, so I tentatively opened the hatch door. From the look on Steve's face, I could tell that the news wasn't good.

'Need you out here, bud. One of the steering lines has snapped.'

Fixing this would be a two-man operation, since we needed to retrieve a new line from the spares bag and get this sorted. It's not such a complex job when you're on a mooring or in calm seas, but in darkness, under extreme tiredness, getting bashed around by waves and swell, wind lashing in our faces and as rain beat down on us, it was an awful lot more tricky.

During the midst of this operation, Steve ended up losing his very good head torch to the depths of the ocean. His response was full of expletives.

Despite the adversity, teamwork conquered all, and eventually the problem was fixed. We could focus once more on our battle to retain first place.

On 20 January, Two-Inna-Row got ahead of us – an inevitability, based on the last few days as we saw them gradually gaining. When it happened it was really bizarre. It was the early hours, and just for a change our GPS wasn't working. Steve was on the oars, and I heard a little commotion outside as I was drifting in and out of sleep.

Steve described it as 'a boat suddenly lighting up out of nowhere'. Sean and Darryl's boat was unique in design – almost futuristic-looking – as it overtook us without warning. They were so close that we were actually able to chat to them over VHF. It was the closest we'd been to actual living, breathing people since leaving La Gomera.

In practice, the 'chat' was more of a shouting contest as we tried to have a conversation over the elements, but it was good to check in on each other and engage with people that were enduring the same experience as us. Despite having been overtaken, we weren't that bothered; we actually quite liked the fact that we'd be the team chasing them down, rather than vice versa.

It gave us some daily targets to aim for, and we were confident that we could catch them again.

A couple of days after this, they had issues with a failed autohelm. They had a much larger and more complicated autohelm system installed on their LB4 vessel. This wasn't likely to be a quick fix for them, and there was the possibility they'd have to steer manually for the rest of the row, or until they fixed the system. As a result, they slowed down, and we were able to reclaim our first position. We hoped that they'd be able to fix it, since we didn't want to win for this reason, and the hard-fought battle was helping to push both of our teams along. To their credit, they were able to get it sorted within 24 hours, and the battle was resumed for first place.

We reached another landmark on 24 January – just 500 miles to go! We duly celebrated with rum on deck. To date, we'd done fairly well with rationing the rum, using it to celebrate positive milestones, as opposed to washing away the setbacks. Come to think of it, that's probably why there was so much left by the time we got to Antigua.

Coming to terms with the fact that I was no Nostradamus, and learning lessons from my previous bold predictions, I called out to Steve, 'Woo-hoo! The final five. How many days do you reckon?'

'I'm enjoying it out here, so hopefully a fair few more,' he replied. 'Besides, I still haven't caught any fish.'

He was quite correct, having invested in a small amount of fishing equipment while in La Gomera, so I was hoping he'd get some sort of nibble.

Regardless, having plenty of rum left meant we could enjoy social drinks on deck a bit more often, so we scheduled in a few more landmarks. Rum night was always fun, and probably more so for whichever one of us had their two-hour sleep shift immediately after.

Another positive was further wildlife encounters, which had been rather lacking for most of our row to date. We put this down to the now limited variety of music available on my iPhone – it would seem the raspy vocals of Bryan Adams were the very opposite of a whale song.

The other ocean life we encountered were more willing to respect our boundaries than the flying fish. There was a close encounter with a pod of dolphins, and we were also tracked for a good few hours by a rather large fish, which we think was a barracuda (we postponed any boat-cleaning activities during this time). Steve had a go at enticing it with his fishing equipment, but to no avail.

After a day of positives, we were soon back to being challenged by our equipment – specifically the autotillers. We'd struggled with these throughout, having already lost two, so we'd been managing with the remaining two for the last couple of weeks, namely Andy and Dave. We'd been taking great care of them, swapping them over very regularly so as to manage their workload. We feared that Dave was on his last legs, and sadly, 30 minutes into his shift, he got so hot that his plastic housing melted. Sorry, Dave.

We continued to manually steer for a few hours, but Steve had already decided to try to resurrect Chris by using spare parts from Dave, and locked himself away in the sweat box of the cabin to start work. While in there, he chatted to a really helpful chap at Raymarine, the autotiller manufacturers, via the satellite phone.

Steve proved to be an absolute master at ocean-based boat repair, combining his practical skills with the feedback and guidance over the phone, and it worked. I don't think I'll ever forget his look of pride as we tested it, and rightly so.

'Petey, Petey!' Steve cried out.

When Steve is excited by something or generally in a good mood, my name suddenly becomes Petey, as opposed to numerous other variations. Therefore, on hearing him call out, I knew he was confident. With Dave's housing melted, Steve had used Chris's housing and transferred various working parts of Dave to Chris. We conducted the usual autotiller swap-over routine, locked on to a bearing and rowed. We both yelled with delight as we realised it was operational – against all odds, Steve had given life to the Atlantic's first zombie autotiller.

Little wins mean an awful lot on the vast ocean, and this meant we could focus on efficiently bringing down the mileage.

'Best day ever,' were my final words to Steve that day as he retired to his quarters.

We couldn't control the elements or other teams' progress, so we chose to focus on the things that we could control: continuing to eat as much as we could to stay physically strong, and doing our best to motivate each other and keep our spirits up. This was just as well, as we were to face another ordeal that would severely test our mood.

The GPS issues that caused our unwelcome close encounter with the boat had continued to plague us.

While we got it up and running for a time, more often than not it would conk out again and lose the satellites.

Around 28 January, while it was in one of its offline phases, we managed to get blown south – further south than Antigua. We were absolutely devastated, since we'd purposely adjusted our bearing from the manual compass in an attempt to compensate for the wind we were cutting through.

It's hard to emphasise the difficulty of rowing while relying on a manual compass – essentially, the compass bearing is not the 'true' bearing. This is because of something called magnetic variance, which marks the difference between the 'magnetic' north and the 'true' north. This can vary over time – it's not such a massive issue on land, say, if you're hiking, as it's usually only out by a couple of degrees.

In the ocean, however, the magnetic variance is a lot bigger, and you have the significant added issue of wind direction, which is a great influence on your direction of travel. This was the main issue for us, since without GPS and a working chartplotter, we just couldn't be sure what our real direction of travel was. Now we were closing in on our target of Antigua, there was simply less margin for error.

On this day, we'd both felt strong, putting everything into our shifts, and were upbeat about the progress we'd made, working off an adjusted bearing on our manual compass to compensate for the crosswinds we were cutting through. We were very confident that we'd maintained the desired westerly direction of travel.

We were absolutely dismayed when we found out from Tim that we'd been blown further south than intended. So much for keeping that little advantage in our back pocket – indeed, the only one we had over Two-Inna-Row. The forecasting from our weather router indicated that we'd be better placed if we were more north on our approach to Antigua, so this was a blow.

Tim had been absent for the previous 24 hours due to attending a wedding, and given that Steve and I had beasted our shifts on the oars, we were keen to catch up with him and see what the next plan of action was. Steve, in good spirits, called him on the satellite phone while I was rowing. 'What? Fucking hell!' I heard Steve say. It was a short call.

I called over to Steve. 'So, the wedding wasn't the best then?' in the hope that Steve's reaction wasn't rowing-related, despite the growing pit in my stomach knowing that it probably was.

'Don't know mate, but Tim's just told me we're now more south than Antigua and just need to focus on getting north again,' Steve said grimly. 'This could literally take days.'

My jaw hit the floor, followed by extensive cursing of the lack of GPS. We were flying blind in terms of knowing our precise direction of travel. Now we were honing in on our target of Antigua, the need for accuracy was becoming critical.

After the Christmas/New Year cabin confinement, this was probably our lowest point. We'd convinced ourselves that we had a chance of getting to Antigua by the end of January or very early February – now, mid-February was looking the more realistic prospect. We also had to focus on getting ourselves further north and cutting back through the wind, with our average daily mileage dropping significantly.

We were both affected mentally by this, now faced with having to prepare ourselves for a further fortnight at sea. It was no problem on the food front (we'd started with enough for 65 days, so had plenty left), but the psychological blow was huge. We'd mentally let ourselves imagine finishing, enjoying home comforts and seeing loved ones. Two more weeks of discomfort wasn't a prospect that we relished.

We both had relatives who were already in Antigua – my dad, and Steve's wife, Corina. We ran the risk of missing them on arrival. Corina had booked a fortnight in Antigua, and there was a real chance that Steve would arrive on the final days of her holiday, or miss her completely.

I was in the same position with my dad. I was on the phone to him, voicing my frustration and apologising to him for this situation and the fact that he'd be kicking his heels in Antigua on his own. His words will stick with me – he simply said, 'I'm here for as long as it takes. I'm incredibly proud of you, and I've got a fridge full of cold beers ready for your arrival. Just stick at it and stay positive.'

Amid all this gloom, there was a brief and very welcome uplift. During one of the few occasions when the GPS and AIS were working, we were able to make contact with a cruise ship, *Ventura*, that we were on a collision course with. Unlike our last close encounter with a large vessel, this was infinitely more controlled, since it happened in the middle of the afternoon, and we were able to reach them instantly on VHF.

Steve had a good chat with the captain and told him what we were doing and how long we had been at sea, as well as encouraging him to share our fundraising link with all the passengers on board.

'Also, would you mind chucking a crate of Heineken overboard for us please?' he asked. Worth a try.

The captain was fascinated with what he heard, and altered course so he could arrange a pass-by at a safe distance, which he announced to the passengers so that they were able to see us.

It was massively uplifting for both of us, and was just the tonic we needed to get ourselves together and make a final push. To hear another human voice and actually see a vessel that we knew was packed with passengers interested in and in disbelief at what we were doing, made a positive difference. It made us both forget our woes and once again reflect on the positives, being that we'd really broken the back of the challenge and to just keep believing.

The cruise ship was still some distance away, but we were told that the passengers could just about make out our vessel. Apparently, this had been the highlight of their cruise to date. Thankfully, they couldn't see our withered, naked Mr Burns-esque bodies from where they were. Might have ruined their holiday.

From a mindset perspective, this encounter was really uplifting, and seemed to do the trick. While 31 January was another slow day, the mileage eventually picked up, pushing us back up to a 50-mile average for the first two days of February.

The morning after marked another milestone: 100 miles to go. The countdown was on.

Interlude 13.1

IN MID-JANUARY, we broke through the 1,000-miles-to-go point, which made the countdown a bit easier and more exciting. The weather was getting warmer by the day, the water seemed to be getting bluer, and the weather was settling.

We were in a routine and knew what we were doing. We still had the daily chores of manually desalinating water, moving meals around the boat to ensure she was trimmed correctly, and were optimising her speed through the water.

Maintenance seemed never-ending: repairing oars, replacing the seat wheel bearings, retying knots on the rudder, trying to turn two broken autotillers into one working one. Cleaning was also an important chore – not just our bodies to keep the saltwater sores at bay, but the boat itself. Everything needed to be spotless. Expedition meal pouches needed to be washed out, dried, folded and stored to prevent rotting, smells and general untidiness. This all took time and effort.

Flying fish are common in these parts, and needed immediate removal from the boat whenever they landed on deck, as they start to decompose almost instantly and smell very bad. Some were the size of my big toe, and others like a small mackerel, about 10in long. The big ones tend to hurt, as they hit you at about 35mph, as Pete found out when one slapped him in the face.

I got hit in the middle of my back during one quiet night on the oars. It comes as quite a shock when you're half asleep, going through the motions in the silence of midnight. When I told Pete about that incident, he asked how I responded. I replied, 'I stamped him to death, called him a c**t, and threw him back in the sea.' This seemed to amuse him for a while.

Equipment became our main concern, and did cause anxiety throughout, more so in the latter third, as parts of our old boat began to show their age and fall apart. Our four autotillers were down to two, and the steering lines were starting to fail. Everything was squeaking and groaning, and we were very conscious of how fragile the boat was. Just one thing breaking could put us back days or even weeks. Having one autotiller would mean foot- or hand-steering, which would really slow us down. Having a very temperamental GPS unit/receiver was already causing issues.

I'd been on the oars mid-afternoon and when we swapped over I went in the cabin but noticed the AIS was beeping to signal a collision course with another vessel. I immediately opened the hatch and looked around. I was alarmed to see a huge cruise ship a few miles from our port side, and quickly tried to reach them on our VHF. Thankfully, they confirmed that they could see us both on the AIS and with the naked eye.

The interactions and conversations with the team on the bridge of the cruise ship became a highlight of the row. We discussed what we were doing, talked about our fundraising targets and charities and tried to encourage the captain to put a Tannoy announcement out to encourage spectators and donations.

The captain said he'd come alongside us, and he tried, but by the time he'd managed to slam the brakes on and do a 90-degree turn, the behemoth was probably about a mile away, so we couldn't see a lot, but when we returned to the UK we caught up with social media and saw that we'd received some messages and photos from passengers of the vessel.

All in all, it was a fantastic 30-minute interaction that still lives with me today – even if we didn't get the case of Heineken we'd asked to be floated over.

Steve Hayes

Interlude 13.2

A FEW weeks after meeting Pete when he started working at Prosperity 24/7, he mentioned in a very quiet way that he liked to do 'a bit of running'. For most of us, this would typically mean five or perhaps ten kilometres, but then Pete's choice of hobbies and adventures are, shall we say, not the same as most of us.

Later, I heard through colleagues that he'd run the Marathon des Sables, a marathon in Greenland, and more. Knowing that he liked a challenge, I brought an article into the office, a piece from *Runner's World* magazine about a particularly challenging Scottish run, which stated 'be warned – people have been brought back in body bags', and I showed the piece to Pete to see his reaction. Casually, he replied that he'd completed that challenge just a few years prior. Well, this was certainly an introduction to the type of person who had just become our CFO – not your usual accountant!

Pete is one of the most humble people I know; humble about his day-to-day financial work at Prosperity, humble about his sporting achievements, humble in everything. He's also one of the most supportive of people when someone else is attempting their own challenge, no matter how much that challenge may pale in comparison to his own. My first attempt at a marathon was London 2020, which unfortunately couldn't go ahead in London itself, and had to take place in Jersey due to Covid restrictions. Pete was there all the way, running parts with us, providing tasty snacks and being there at the makeshift finish line with handmade medals for me and my friend Rose, with London-themed pressies to congratulate us.

There are two challenges in particular that stick in my mind as being almost superhuman: firstly, Pete choosing to pull a car over a marathon distance in Jersey, and then, of course, the Atlantic Row.

I still can't get my head around why someone would choose to pull a car, but to then go on and row the Atlantic distance is even more (quite literally) incredible.

Alongside the physicality of these challenges are the enormous efforts that go into his fundraising. His Atlantic row involved around 18 months of administration, and conversations with – and securing sponsorship from – corporates and the wider community.

The commitment to get physically fit for this type of challenge is no mean feat. I felt physically sick thinking of Pete and Steve out on the water for that duration, and in those conditions – to such a degree that I found it very difficult to talk to Pete about it at work without breaking into a sweat! I remember Pete calling me on a satellite phone from the race when, due to strong winds, they'd been blown the wrong direction. Despite this awful situation, he was still upbeat and positive. It was me who needed a brandy to settle my nerves, having heard a little of what he'd been through and what he had still to do to complete the challenge!

But with Pete, you realise that there's a lot more to this quiet accountant. He loves the outdoors, he loves to be challenged and to push himself, and most of all he loves his community and raising much-needed funds for charities that are close to his heart.

Geraldine Evans, co-founder, Prosperity 24/7,
Pete's employers

Chapter 14

Cool runnings

THE ICE Ultra. It takes place in Swedish Lapland across 230km and five days of seemingly unending icy wilderness in and around the Arctic Circle, and is often described as the world's last wilderness.

Along the way are frozen lakes, glaciers, and other natural phenomena that fall firmly into the 'off the beaten track' category. There are no coffee stops; self-sufficiency is the name of the game here, so everything you need has to be carried with you on your back.

An incredibly long distance taking place over one of the most inhospitable environments the world has to offer. To successfully complete this, two things would be key: preparation and a high level of physical fitness.

I was probably the most physically unprepared I had ever been. The lead-up to this race had been a complete and utter nightmare, thanks to my mum's cancer diagnosis and the subsequent inexplicably hostile behaviour of my then-boss (see Chapter 16 for a more detailed account of this). However, this is a positive book, and I won't waste ink on people for whom I'd have a carefully chosen description if asked.

While exercise is a good outlet in times of stress, it can't be underestimated just how much the latter can seriously impact the former. The mental toll of these last few months had serious ramifications for my fitness. Physically, I was the most unfit I'd been in years – my whole body seemed locked up with stress. I needed two sports massages in the week before the event to ensure I could just straighten my back.

Despite all of this, I was determined to get to the start line. It was all paid for, and a mini-break facing the elements was just what I needed. My work predicament was not going to change unless I instigated it. I felt confident that this trip would be the start of the process.

In the lead-up to the race, I'd been part of a Facebook group with other competitors, and had arranged to meet one of these, Simon Davies, at Gatwick. We established a firm friendship in no time at all, and I instantly felt refreshed by his positive company. We headed to the departures lounge for our flight to Luleå in Sweden, where we were met by two other competitors, Aaron Trindall and Andrew Wicking. Both had suffered DNFs at the previous year's Ice Ultra, and were back for a second attempt.

These DNFs were linked to the extremities we'd be facing during this race. Now, the nerves were kicking in, since I hadn't really considered the possibility of a DNF. This race was supposed to be a first step to rebuilding some self-esteem, so a momentary thought of failure was a sobering one. I put that out of my head as soon as I could, and resolved to complete this event, one way or another.

The following day, we boarded a small train to Gällivare, and met a few more competitors. Once there, it was on to base camp and a three-hour coach trip. It seemed to be a good group, and in no time there was banter between the competitors, race crew and medical team.

We'd barely set foot in base camp when the mandatory checks began, starting with kit. These were probably the most thorough I'd ever experienced, and considering what we'd be facing, it was no surprise – frostbite and hypothermia were very real risks, and were the primary reason for competitors not completing the race. I'd researched my kit well and had the opportunity to test a great deal of it in Finnish Lapland the previous December while on holiday with Rachel and the kids.

Once all the mandatory checks were done, it was time to chill, eat and get ready for an introductory first night sleeping in an outdoor tepee in a thermal sleeping bag with a thermal liner. With the conditions as they were, it was a cold, uncomfortable night. It was the pre-race nerves that kept me awake, rather than the weather, though. I was still undecided on how exactly I was going to dress, and wanted to guard against being too layered up on account of generating excess sweat, which wouldn't be good. I'd pretty much decided that it would be a thermal base layer and a down jacket, but I was wondering whether I needed to add more. There were lots of 'what ifs' flying around my head, firmly driven by the unknown. These types of thoughts and general apprehension of the unknown contributed to the lack of sleep on this night.

Day 1: Circumnavigating Mount Kabla

Wake-up was 5am for a 7am start. I mostly slept in my kit, so final preparations consisted of a dash to the toilets to apply the finishing touches, before heading off to a communal hut for some rehydrated granola (don't knock it 'til you've tried it).

By now, nervous tension was rife among all the competitors – we all just wanted to get going. With the race start impending, I fastened my snowshoes to my trail running shoes. I took great care, ensuring the straps were fastened tight, since I didn't want to be making any adjustments once the race got going – or worse, see them falling off. Extreme cold and thick gloves make adjustments tricky. As if to prove my point, I saw a fellow competitor's snowshoes fall off just as the race commenced. Not ideal. It took him a good few minutes to sort them out and get moving again.

It was the first time I'd used the snowshoes, and they took some getting used to. Frustratingly, a delay in postage meant I didn't have them to practise in for my earlier trip to Finland, and Jersey doesn't exactly get flurries of snow. My best alternative was to use them a little on the sand dunes in Jersey, but I was mindful that sand is heavier and denser than snow, and I didn't want to damage them.

On race start, I felt clumsy and ungainly as I got used to them, but quickly adapted. I'd also started off in snow goggles, but found my vision far too restricted, so I stashed these away and stuck with sunglasses. The goggles would be strictly for blizzard use.

As for the rest of my attire, I had a Brynje Arctic layer and a Jöttnar shell for my top half, and another couple of layers for the bottom half. The two-layer approach was retained for my hands, being liner gloves and shell gloves, along with a good beanie hat and a buff. I ensured the hat covered the tips of my ears, and would pull the buff up over my nose from time to time – both anti-frostbite measures. I was genuinely worried that my massive hooter would attract frostbite at some point, so was fairly religious about pulling my buff over my face from time to time. My outfit was finished off by liner socks with thermal socks over the top – plus the trail shoes and snowshoes, obviously.

First impressions were how tough it was underfoot, and the difficulty in regulating breathing in the unfamiliar cold climate. I definitely wasn't at all 'running fit' heading into this one, the energy I was expending trying to quicken my pace becoming apparent. To make things easier for myself, I started walking and running at intervals, slowly increasing the latter as I went along. On the plus side, my body temperature felt fine, and I wasn't cold but also wasn't overly sweating.

Before I knew it, I'd reached checkpoint one. It sounds obvious, but it's always a nice milestone, since you know you're officially in a race, and those following your movements online can see your progress as your race tracker bleeps through the first milestone. I'd made a conscious effort to drink regularly, so I refilled my bottles and moved on quickly. Doing this was key – not only to stay hydrated, but also to stop the liquid and nozzles from freezing.

While I stuck to this plan to begin with, I lapsed into bad habits on the way to the second checkpoint.

All it took was 15 minutes of hydration inaction – upon raising the bottle to my lips, I found it frozen solid. Luckily, by this point, I was close to the second checkpoint, and the race crew were on hand to thaw it out. The checkpoints were generally tepees with a cauldron of boiling water in the centre, so thawing out the bottle was easy enough.

'Ah, another one,' exclaimed the medic as I trudged in almost apologetically, holding out my soft flask.

'Yep. Didn't take long,' I replied.

'Just drink every five minutes and keep squashing and shaking the bottle,' was the advice offered, and I resolved to do this from now on. Lesson learned. I'd now be using my bottles every five minutes without fail.

Meanwhile, my food strategy was working. I was mindful of foods that would freeze or harden, and for checkpoints I'd invested in noodles. I basically had an empty foil bag (from an old expedition meal) in which I'd put my noodles and add hot water at each checkpoint. Noodles were easy enough to consume, and settled well in the stomach. I'd read some blogs from previous competitors, and they were very much recommended.

On leaving checkpoint four, I felt a pain on my foot, originating from the strapping of the snowshoe. The conditions seemed firm and generally okay, so I decided to remove the snowshoes and just run in my trail shoes. I also thought this would assist me in terms of speed. This didn't really work – as soon as I hit the inevitable deeper snow, I started to sink. I hadn't fully appreciated the snowshoes' capacity and value to act like miniature skis, effectively stopping you from sinking in the snow and wasting valuable energy.

Realising my mistake, I tried to put the snowshoes back on, but by this point the straps had hardened due to the conditions and had little flexibility, so I couldn't get them tight enough. Left with no other choice, I strapped them to the back of my race pack and moved on, cursing my indecision and stupid mistake in such an inhospitable environment.

Incidentally, the cause of the pain turned out to be a series of solid icicles formed on the inside of the strapping that were digging into the top of my foot, which I noticed while trying to put them back on – that's the Arctic for you!

I didn't see another soul for the rest of the day, and it proved to be a long, hard slog to the finish. That said, I was loving it. This environment, even though harsh, was absolutely stunning, and very peaceful. I felt lucky to be here.

On arrival into camp, I was directed to the main cabin, where most other competitors were. It was chaos, with kit explosions everywhere. I was in the bottom third in terms of positioning, so there was literally no room left. It was absolute bedlam in there, as competitors were rushing around, and there were clearly no more beds. I made my way back over the road, and was invited to join the crew and medics' cabin, which was warm and accommodating. In fact, I probably got the better deal, since this cabin was much nicer. My lack of training had really paid off!

I had a good chat with Kris King, the race director, and got to witness the hectic life of an RD as he made call after call. Our conversation was fairly stop-start on account of all the issues that were arising. Kris told me a little about the history of the race and the close relationship his team had formed with the Sámi people, who had allowed this race to take place in their territory. The firm objective of Kris and his team that evening – and every other – was to ensure the safe arrival of everyone into camp. Once this was achieved, his focus switched to the logistics of the following day. Even while I slept, I could hear Kris dealing with various issues. It had been a tough day for many, for one reason or another. There had been a few DNFs, mainly thanks to frostbite.

Happily, I wasn't counted among their number – I didn't even have any feet issues, which had to be a first. I had plenty of time to chill out, dry my damp clothes, eat and get my bag packed for the following day. By 10pm, I was sound asleep.

Day 2: Climbing Mount Kabla

Today was my 45th birthday, and what a way to spend it.

I'd finished the previous day in the dark, and had little idea of the natural beauty that surrounded me. As I left the cabin, I was greeted by a stunning view of the mountains and a clear blue sky. It definitely beat a morning run across the local housing estate.

I resolved to start the race in snowshoes and avoid any temptation to remove them. This was particularly important today, as the race briefing warned us that it would be particularly cold, with temperatures forecast to go as low as minus 45°C. I had no idea what that type of temperature would even feel like – apart from bloody cold, obviously – so I paid special attention to my admin and layering options that morning.

I decided to adopt the same kit strategy as the previous day, but did wonder whether my hands would be sufficiently protected by the tried-and-trusted two-layer system. Sure enough, five minutes in, I could feel my fingertips biting. It was a certain kind: one that was not going to get any better.

This prompted an early decision to retrieve my Arctic mittens – easier said than done, since my hands had already frozen rigid, making getting into my pack a monumental challenge. However, once the job was done, I was on my way. The Arctic mittens were absolute beasts, keeping my digits safely toasty. However, the downside is that they left my hands resembling ungainly crab claws, meaning it wasn't very easy to retrieve snacks and things like that.

The next 45 minutes on my approach to checkpoint one were spent worrying about frostbite – Kris's late-night overheard bedtime stories on the subject didn't make for fun listening, and my fingertips felt very sore. Thankfully, the pain subsided post-checkpoint. Another lesson learned.

Before I left the first checkpoint, a medic remarked on something I hadn't considered: my face was looking pretty red – not something you'd tend to associate with extreme cold, but it was an issue, all the same! I realised that I'd forgotten to put suntan lotion on – it was still in my camp bag. Out came my Arctic hood for some additional face protection for the day.

The route to checkpoint two saw me move swiftly across a nice flat lake, then onwards to a stunning ascent through a forest and checkpoint two. It was perfect wilderness – the occasional snowmobile zoomed past, driven by someone connected to the race, reminding me what I was here for.

To my surprise, at checkpoint two, Simon Davies came in just behind me. I thought he was well ahead of me, but it turned out he'd taken a wrong turn, costing him an extra 6km. Unsurprisingly, he was raging – all I could do to placate him was remind him that he was looking strong, and should easily be able to make up the ground.

An inconvenient toilet trip – let's call it a special sit-down birthday treat – meant that I'd missed the race briefing for today's stage, so I didn't really have any concept of the distances between checkpoints. In the event, most of my journeys passed by without incident – I simply enjoyed the view and this unique isolated environment. It was bloody cold, though, and daylight was running out, which meant temperatures were going to plummet further. I knew I needed to get a move on to try to finish before it got much colder.

By the time I reached checkpoint five, I was absolutely beasted. It was dark and really cold – minus 45°C cold.

Here was the state of play: there were still 9km left. If skin was exposed to the cold for too long, it became painful. The heavy-duty mittens and balaclava had proved their worth.

Every one of those 9km was a huge challenge. The snowshoes remained, but the ground was now harder underfoot. Hot spots were developing on the bases of my feet.

To quote Rik Mayall in *Bottom*, happy birthday to me!

I've never in all my life experienced cold like that night. Thank god I fuelled up on warm noodles at checkpoint four!

Will Roberts, who was a key member of the race crew, was there to greet me as I slogged into the warm shelter of camp, lifting my spirits immediately when he told me that Rach had posted a message on the race's Instagram: 'Wishing Peteloaf a happy birthday'. That brought a smile to my face.

To cap things off, Simon stuck a candle in a flapjack for me and led a chorus of 'Happy Birthday' from some of the other competitors. It remains one of my all-time favourite birthday cakes.

Before heading to bed, I checked the route for day three. It was to be a similar distance – less cold, but flat and very hard underfoot – and would involve a very long lake crossing. I decided that it was time to try crampons instead of my snowshoes on the basis that I thought I'd be able to move more swiftly. I was very confident that this decision would be the right one, and Simon was of the same opinion.

Sleep arrived quickly that night as I shared a cabin with Simon, Katie Baker and Louis Supple. Katie and Louis both lived in the UK, and loved the outdoor life. We all had a chat and this type of environment in terms of racing was a first for all of us, but we were all in agreement that we were loving it. Lights were out and we were all sleeping soundly once we'd sorted our kit, which is just as well, as the following day wouldn't be easy.

Day 3: Marathon over frozen lakes

Since it had been very cold overnight, crampons felt sufficient. Having made all my errors on previous days, I felt like I was getting used to the environment now, and felt more confident about my decision-making process when it came to things like kit. The only nagging doubt was my swollen feet and how cold they felt. I couldn't believe how much they'd swollen. I made constant efforts to wiggle my toes so I could feel them and keep the circulation going.

I had my usual noodles at checkpoint two – there was always good banter with medics and fellow competitors at the checkpoints, and we were really looked after. From then on, we were faced with long flat marches across lakes. I'd been warned to expect the temperatures to drop again, so had everything I'd need to hand.

In the event, it was very sunny, which took the edge off things. It was only when you pulled your trousers down to go to the toilet that you realised how cold it was – I was always very careful to tuck the old chap in afterwards, lest frostbite threatened to cut him down to size. There were regular flags to mark the route, so I adopted a tactic of running to every other flag to break up the monotony, although the pain in my knees, owing to the very hard ground, kept me alert.

It was a clear day – so much so that you could often see the checkpoints as much as an hour before you actually got there. Then, the sun fell, and darkness came. I could see head torches ahead of me, gradually fading as they finished the stage. It gave me a target to aim for, and I was trying to imagine what today's camp would be like – probably not as luxurious as the previous day's.

For the final hour, I could see no torches ahead of me, and could make out nothing behind me. The only reassuring thing was the flags indicating that I was on the correct route, but I just didn't know how long for. I'd opted to do this race without any form of GPS watch, so never really had an idea on distance travelled unless I asked another competitor or one of the medics at the checkpoints.

Ultimately, the finish seemed to pop out from nowhere. Instant elation.

The cabin I shared with Tony Mather and Simon had a lovely log burner. I'd spent a bit of time with Tony during previous stages. He was a few years older than me, and had a similar passion for anything endurance-related when time allowed outside of family and work. Someone – I can't remember who – had the bright idea of shutting the door in an effort to warm the cabin, which worked in no time, given its small size. However, with only a couple of tiny windows that you could just about put your arm through, it quickly started to get really hot. We'd gone from one extreme to another. We then discovered that the door had frozen shut, and we couldn't get out from the inside. Trapped, and with temperatures soaring, we all had to strip down to our underwear. It felt odd that I was facing an untimely end via extreme heat, as opposed to cold.

My internal voices were having a running battle: *How am I going to explain this one to Rach?* said one. *You won't have to, on account of being dead. Kris King will have to do it*, said the other. Shades of Rik in *The Young Ones* after he accidentally kills Neil.

I chuckled at the thought, only to be caught by Tony glaring with a look that had 'what the fuck are you laughing at?' written all over it.

Fortunately, Kris was saved the job of reporting our untimely demises to our next of kins. After much frantic pushing, we managed to barge our way out. The door remained wedged ajar for the remainder of the night.

The three of us all had a laugh about the episode. The grim reaper tentatively poking his scythe through the door had well and truly put to bed any nerves about the following day's stage.

Before long, snoring was rife – either that or there was an earthquake hitting that very specific region of Sweden. Tony was the guilty party. That, combined with our cabin-bound misadventures, meant that I approached day four armed with very little in the way of sleep.

Day 4: The long day – 65km

I felt genuinely chuffed to still be in this race. The build-up had tested me more than I realised. However, in the three days I'd completed, I had time to reflect on everything, often in a white wilderness where I couldn't hear a sound. It was very therapeutic, and the conclusion I reached was that I'd lost control, and had to take back control when I returned home with regards to the work situation. The solution was simple, so quite why it took me to be freezing my bits off in the Arctic to realise it, I don't know. Plan duly formed, it was time to crack on and get this challenge completed.

While I hadn't really physically prepared for this, I now effectively had three days of solid training under my belt. I was very much training as I went along, definitely getting stronger by the day, and the positivity of the mind was driving the body on.

Still in my crampons, I stuck with my strategy of alternating between running and walking, although now I was doing more of the former. Thus far, I'd drifted to the back of the pack reasonably quickly, resulting in long, isolated days. I knew I wasn't at all 'running fit', so when you combine that with trying to move in alien terrain with equipment I'd never tried out before and a heavy race pack, that I found it tough wasn't a surprise. However, this worked to my advantage, since I'd managed to get my head straightened out. Today, I got off to a much better start, staying in the company of others for longer than usual. This was uplifting.

With multiday racing events, I've always joked that you can train as you go along. This is always advice that you'll find me dishing out to others. However, I was really having to put this into practice on the Ice Ultra. It was easier said than done, but not impossible.

I spent a good amount of time with Simon and Jeff Jeff (yes, that's his name) on the way to checkpoint two, and we were facing some good, manageable terrain. Jeff Jeff was a great guy from Malaysia, and I never saw him without a smile on his face. He was very small in stature, meaning his pack looked gigantic on him, but he was doing really well.

By checkpoint three I was tiring, so earmarked this as a noodle stop. Despite my lack of pace, I was reassured by the fact that I was well ahead of race cut-offs, and was keeping things simple and sensible, having a steady eating strategy and just ticking off each checkpoint at a time.

Checkpoint four was really tough. I felt like I was starting to ration my food too much. It seemed better to save food for later stages, and I wanted noodles again at checkpoint four, but decided to wait for checkpoint five. I didn't usually feel so hungry during races, but there seemed to be something about the Arctic that made me absolutely ravenous.

The next couple of stages went quicker than expected, and it was just getting dark as I arrived at checkpoint six. The terrain had changed significantly, and there were quite a few steep climbs before a kind descent into checkpoint six. Here, I got it into my head that it would be a bit of a jaunt, considering that it was only 8.5km to the end. I couldn't have been more wrong.

After the first kilometre, I saw markings for a right turn. I'd kept my crampons on in the expectation that it would be a hop and a skip to the finish line. Not quite. Here, I was met by very deep, knee-sinking snow with narrow paths and lots of ups and downs. It was dark, and I was extremely tired, disorientated, falling over frequently and desperately trying to follow the markings and not get myself lost. It was incredibly energy-sapping both physically and mentally. Despite being so close to the end, I felt incredibly low. I was cold, tired and extremely hungry. It had been a long day, and it had all caught up with me very quickly.

Everywhere was dark, and I couldn't see any signs of civilisation – not even a reassuring flicker of light or distant voices. I'd expected to hear or see something, since I figured I must be close to the end, and the fact I couldn't added to my anxiety. Was I lost? I couldn't be.

I consoled myself with the fact that I must only be two or three miles from the finish, and tried to equate that to a familiar run I did back home in Jersey. I almost tried to visualise myself being somewhere else, and it seemed to help the situation for a time.

Out of nowhere I saw lights – relief and delight flooded me in equal measure. I sank to my knees and screamed an almighty 'whoo hoo!' Excitement swiftly replaced anxiety.

Will was there to meet me at the finish, and asked if I'd mind a quick interview for their social media channel. I happily obliged, knowing Rach and the kids would be able to see that I was okay and in good spirits.

At one point I said, 'It was a brilliant feeling to get the race done,' to which Will quickly replied, 'You do know there's another stage tomorrow, right?'

I did, of course, but the following day's stage was relatively short in comparison to what we'd faced, and the terrain would be an awful lot kinder as we approached the town we'd finish in.

After the interview, I was directed to a building where we'd be staying. It would be a communal arrangement with sleeping bags on the floor, but it was dry and warm. Sleep came very easily that night, helped by the quiet satisfaction of what had been achieved over the previous four days.

The following day was to be the final and easiest day in terms of distance and what we'd be dealing with. This added to the satisfaction as I drifted into sleep, since I knew I'd all but completed the race.

Day 5: The final 15km to Jokkmokk

I was made aware that the first 6.5km would be over the deep, soft snow that I'd traversed towards the end of the previous day's stage, which I hadn't quite expected. With this news, the snowshoes went back on, but at least I'd be doing this in daylight as opposed to darkness. From here, the final 8.5km would be pretty flat and manageable as we approached the town where the race would finish.

It made complete sense to start with snowshoes first, given my sinking the day before, and then remove these at a checkpoint and go with trail shoes. I probably wouldn't even need crampons, based on the reports I'd seen.

As soon as I started, I realised that I probably didn't really need snowshoes either, since the ground had hardened overnight significantly. However, the night before remained fresh in my mind, so I used them regardless. They weren't hindering my progress.

At checkpoint one, I removed my snowshoes as planned, strapped them to my pack, and went off in trail shoes. My pack was as light as it had been, since I'd gradually been eating all my food. It was now far easier to run a bit quicker, and I resolved to finish the race in style.

From checkpoint one, I was running at a similar pace to Katy and Tony. As I ran, I was now seeing more residents of the fast-approaching town. Civilisation beckoned.

About 3km from the finish, a load of huskie riders shot past, telling me how crazy they thought I was in relation to where we'd run from five days before. Guess they had a point!

The finish came far quicker than I thought, since I figured that there were another 2km to go. I didn't have a GPS watch for this one, so I was just using a basic wristwatch. I guess I'd moved pretty quickly today.

I don't always use my Garmin on multiday events, unless serious navigation is involved, or the course isn't well marked. I sometimes find it's nice just to switch off and enjoy the moment without getting hung up about pacing and splits. This event proved to be one of these occasions, and meant I was looking at things around me rather than getting overly obsessed with data or splits.

The finish was absolutely amazing. I ran over the finish line, and with a big, beaming smile, punched the air and shouted, 'Yes!' Emotions took over a little. I bent down to remove something from my eye, then spotted Simon, so I hugged it out with him. I was greeted by the race team, medics, and fellow competitors who had finished before me. There was a pile of beers in the snow waiting for all of us, and also plenty of hugs.

I hung around outside at the finish with others enjoying an ice-cold beer in the ice-cold, and cheering my fellow competitors as they completed their race. There was so much excitable chatter, and I couldn't help but reflect on what an absolutely amazing experience it had been. After 30 minutes or so, I went inside to get warm and put on some dry clothes – and, of course, drink a couple more well-earned beers.

When everyone was safely in, we boarded a coach to take us to our cabins. I had a lovely warm shower, and chilled with Simon and Tony. Then it was off to the afterparty, where I got to have a good chat with Wolfgang Schönegger, who had also competed in this race. I'd first met him in the Amazon in 2015, and this event had brought us together once again, so it was really nice to see him.

We spoke about what we'd been doing since the jungle. Unsurprisingly, Wolfgang had been taking on gnarly races regularly, either in his native Germany or somewhere else globally. I'd seen him on a few occasions during the race, as he always overtook me with the aid of his trusty stick. I think he'd found it on day one, and 'Wolfgang's stick' became quite notorious by the end.

The afterparty beckoned in good food, great company, great beers and a few Jägers. What an event, and what a night.

The following day's coach journey back to civilisation probably required the most endurance of the whole week, as I battled a rather suspect alcohol-induced hangover, and sleep deprivation once again brought on by Tony's snoring.

I'd done it: the Ice Ultra was conquered, and I'd well and truly renewed my focus. That's one of the great things about these kinds of challenges: you put yourself through the mill, and at the other end you seem to know yourself better.

The challenge of my situation at work hadn't changed, but I seemed better equipped for how to deal with it. There were many times during this race where I was on my own, and I just looked around at the snow-covered wilderness and simply reflected. It was like looking at a blank canvas, and I now had the opportunity to change the narrative and get started on a new story. I headed home, excited to see Rach and the kids again, and equally excited to settle some scores.

Interlude 14

I FIRST met Pete during the BTU Ice Ultra. It's a race that tests every ounce of your endurance, and typical of the sort of challenge Pete regularly takes in his stride. Pete and I seemed to settle into the same pace from the start. We didn't talk much – the Arctic cold has a way of stealing your breath and freezing any spare words mid-air. But his steady company was reassuring – a reminder that neither of us was truly alone out there.

On the third evening of the race, after hours of endless snow and biting wind, we reached a small fishing hut on a frozen lake. It was supposed to be a refuge, but 'primitive' doesn't quite cover it. The place was a wooden box barely holding back the cold, with frost creeping along the walls.

Pete took over the stove, bringing it to life. The fire was a welcome distraction, and for a while the room transformed into a cosy escape. We eagerly peeled off layers of frozen gear and let the warmth seep in. But then the stove started to overdeliver. The fire roared, filling the tiny space with unbearable heat. What had been our salvation quickly became a serious threat.

The door, swollen from the sudden rise in temperature, wouldn't budge. Pete and I exchanged a look, neither of us panicked, but both keenly aware of the problem. The air grew thick, each breath shallow and strained as sweat poured off us. The irony wasn't lost on us – here we were, trained and dressed for freezing temperatures, now trying not to dangerously overheat in the middle of the Arctic.

After several failed attempts to force the door, we stripped right down to our underwear and braced ourselves for one final push. With a combination of brute force and determination, the door finally gave way. The frigid air hit us like a wall, but it was a relief.

We stumbled outside and fell into the snow, the icy ground cooling us instantly. Lying there in the minus 40°C night, steam rising from our red, sweating and overheated bodies, we laughed with relief. The biting cold stung against our skin, but it was an incredible feeling.

That moment from the Ice Ultra stuck with me. Pete's calmness under pressure and his ability to keep things in perspective were exactly what you needed in a place as unforgiving as the Arctic. Sharing an adventure like that with Pete wasn't just about surviving the race – it was a lesson in resilience, steady resolve and good humour. Pete's traits weren't just admirable, they were a reminder of what it means to face challenges with determination and composure.

Pete's not just a great athlete, but the kind of person you always want to have in your corner.

Simon Davies, friend and fellow
ultramarathon runner

Chapter 15

(Budgie) smugglers
of the Caribbean

WITH 100 miles to go, we decided to just go for it. Our recent progress had pushed our arrival time well down again – at one point we were predicted to get in early on 15 February; now, we could be in as early as the 5th. Game on.

Our preference, however, was to get in on the evening of Saturday, 4th. By this point, Two-Inna-Row were well ahead of us, with little prospect of us catching them up. Our predicament a few days earlier – when we were blown more south than Antigua, and then had to spend the next day rowing north – had cost us in our race against them. We'd been advised that it would take us days to recover our previous position, but we both embraced this as a challenge, sacrificed some sleep and managed to recover our position in a single day. This single day was enough to put our opponents a good 30 miles ahead of us. Now, with that out of our minds, we were rowing our own race, and we wanted to finish strongly.

We had a discussion around when we were likely to finish, and what we could realistically do to influence this. The probability seemed high that we'd finish in the early hours of Sunday, and we both didn't really want this. Ideally, we wanted to arrive in the evening or during daylight hours, on the basis that there may be a few people to see us in. We both agreed that it would be impossible to force a slowdown, and just wouldn't be the right way to finish a race. With this in mind, we just agreed to hit the hammer and try to get in Saturday evening.

The conditions, as Tim had predicted, seemed to be turning in our favour, each two-hour rowing shift feeling really productive. As an added bonus, the GPS and chartplotter had come back to life, and we had full visibility of our nautical mileage and position. It was also a time for reflection – since the mileage was going down, we began to realise that we were approaching several 'lasts': last sunrise, last sunset, last poo in the bucket. The list went on.

Everything seemed to be happening in stages – Steve was the first to catch sight of dry land as I was completing my rowing shift. He told me as soon as he spotted land, but I told him I wanted to wait until I'd finished my rowing shift, so that I had something to look forward to.

The moment came, and Steve had the GoPro out to record the moment.

He called out, 'Here we are … Petey about to see land for the first time in 50 days.' With that, I stood up and turned to my side for Steve to say, 'Oh, where's it gone? It was there a minute ago.' The position of the sun was obscuring things now.

I craned my neck – finally, land! It was an absolutely amazing sight. It was also a time to reflect on the huge distance we'd covered. We could actually see our target, which just seemed to spur us on, with a celebratory rum being our reward. That said, we'd come to learn that the ocean was a rather unpredictable friend, and we couldn't take anything for granted in our approach.

Even so, in true DragonFish style, we found time for some mishaps. Somehow, I managed to drop my phone – one of our few working devices – on the deck, instantly shattering half of the screen. It was now unusable, meaning we had no music to listen to, or Wi-Fi for WhatsApp communications – just the satellite phone and our VHF radio. Thankfully, Steve kept his harmonica stowed away.

With the conditions in our favour and the wind on our tail, we went without sleep in an attempt to get in quicker. This worked out well, as we managed to cover 64 miles on the penultimate day. The ability to see land, have working GPS and therefore the ability to see what speed we were rowing, really spurred us on, and positivity of progress was certainly breeding positivity of the mind. My backside suddenly didn't feel sore anymore, and I felt energised. Each rowing shift seemed to go really quickly and we really felt we were working with the ocean in a very positive way. The Atlantic was now flirting with us, as opposed to being a cruel mistress. Knowing that we could rest properly once we were in Antigua, we put everything into it.

Coming into the last day, we crossed over into the Caribbean tectonic plate. This marked a big difference: previously, the depth of the water we rowed across could have been anywhere between 4,000 and 6,000ft. Now, it was just a couple of hundred. The ocean felt different at this point. For the majority of the row, the energy that moves around the ocean had plenty of space to do so, which quite often resulted in big, long rollercoaster swells. Now that the energy was compressed into a smaller space, the waves felt sharper and far more choppy.

While it was very tempting to team up and row together in order to cross the line more quickly, ultimately we decided against this. We were used to rowing by ourselves, and had developed our own methods. When we tried rowing together, it was the first time we'd attempted this in a while, and it showed, resulting in plenty of clashing – both between the oars and ourselves as the frustration grew. This approach proving counter-productive, we quickly agreed that it was best to row solo.

With the end getting nearer, we had a brief heart-to-heart moment. A bit soppy, maybe, but we were chuffed with ourselves that we'd managed to get to this point. I told Steve it had been an absolute honour to have this experience with him, and couldn't really have imagined doing it with anyone else. I added that he was 'like a brother to me', and we subsequently hugged it out.

Before we'd even set off on the row, we'd explain to people the anticipated challenge of living with anyone for over 50 days, let alone in a space the size of a boardroom table (and with that person naked for an ample proportion of that time). I remember Steve often telling people, when asked, that he couldn't imagine 50 days alone with his wife, let alone someone else (Corina, if you're reading this, I'm almost entirely sure that he was joking).

We also didn't really know what versions of ourselves we'd become, but always promised to find various techniques that would simply get the best out of each other. This would depend on our moods, and could involve a friendly joke, a stern talking-to or simply a squeeze of the shoulder or a hug. The row had made our already strong friendship even stronger. We'd nailed it, and to genuinely enjoy the experience with someone meant far more to me than a quicker time of finishing in first place.

Still, we weren't out of the woods just yet. Approaching Antigua, we enjoyed our final sunset. It was soon incredibly dark, and our final waypoint ran its course. At this point, we really weren't sure on our approach to Antigua. Having called Ian Couch to get approach directions, we were told to follow the headland and look for an inlet, where a support boat would be waiting to guide us in. With our GPS operational, I entered the cabin and monitored the chartplotter as the final rowing shift began.

As odd as it sounds, navigationally this was probably the trickiest part of the journey. Before, we were in a vast expanse and heading in the rough direction of Antigua, with no hazards to worry about, such as rocks or land. Now, we were in unfamiliar territory and clearly not used to navigating hazards.

We also needed to ensure that we didn't miss the entrance into English Harbour (the port town where the race ended) – the wind was firmly on our tail, and we were rocketing in. This presented a very real risk that we could actually be swept past the entrance to the harbour at great speed, so I was taking great care looking at the chartplotter and shouting instructions to Steve. It was like trying to find a pinprick in the dark.

We finally caught sight of the lights from the support boat, and could now see the entrance into the harbour. I came out of the cabin and grabbed both steering lines. It would now be my job to steer while Steve rowed through the toughest conditions he'd experienced to date. He rowed hell for leather, against the fiercest of crosswinds. We thought about swapping over, but with approach conditions as chaotic as they were, it was best to just stick as we were and focus on getting into that harbour. Once we were in, we'd have shelter, and that would be that.

Of course, we had to make sure we were dressed for the occasion – and the occasion called for speedos, emblazoned with the DragonFish logo.

Steve had gone to great care in ordering these, so I couldn't let him down. Finally, my hair clippers came in useful, since we both took the opportunity to shave further down in an effort to look tidy when we came in. Considering the amount of time we – especially Steve – spent in a state of undress, a pair of speedos was quite conservative attire.

As we entered the port of English Harbour, we were suddenly approached by a couple of ribs, both crewed by Atlantic Campaigns – one to guide us in, and the other to collect our passports and all SD cards. This was standard stuff, apparently – Atlantic Campaigns need them to review and identify any possible evidence of a rule breach.

As we prepared to cross the finish line, we got the flares out. Knowing that I couldn't be trusted with anything fire-related after my disastrous attempt to light a match at Cubs, Steve lit mine for me.

The final few strokes were upon us, Steve was rowing his heart out and the guy on the support boat was screaming out a countdown of ten down to one on our approach to the finish line.

Finally, we crossed – instant euphoria! Two years of planning, preparation, ups and downs, introspection and nerves, culminated in this moment. It was a head to the sky moment, desperately trying to take in what we'd just achieved.

Just before midnight on Saturday, 4 February 2023, having set off on 12 December 2022, we completed our journey in 54 days. We'd done it: we'd completed the toughest row in the world.

As we held our flares, we screamed and shouted with absolute joy. I had to drop my flare into the Richard III bucket after about a minute, as it was bloody hot (I must have been holding it too high up – how utterly predictable, given my track record with fire).

This didn't dampen my euphoric mood, though, and I was happy enough to punch the air in delight while keeping hold of the side of the boat, as my legs felt pretty unsteady. We looked around at English Harbour. For the first time in almost two months, we were about to hit dry land and see other human beings. I desperately wanted to see Rachel and the kids at this point, but I consoled myself with the thought that they'd be watching on the live feed.

Rachel was a couple of weeks away from an operation for her brain aneurysm. This was news that I'd found out mid-row, and the date of operation was to be my 50th birthday on 21 February. Josh also had his mock exams fast approaching, so we'd all agreed that an in-person greeting in Antigua wouldn't be possible.

My dad had surprised me mid-row when he told me on the satellite phone that he'd be there to see me in. I was close to tears when I heard this, since I honestly believed I wouldn't have anyone there. However, as our anticipated arrival time bounced around in the final fortnight, I did feel very guilty that he'd needed to extend his stay on the island. He was happy enough, though, immersing himself in the rowing community and studying the local wildlife.

Steve's wife Corina and his daughter Sophia had also been on the island the same time as my dad. Poor old Steve had worried that he'd have no time with them in Antigua, but as it turned out he had a week with them.

As we rowed in alongside the pier, we were pleasantly surprised to see a large crowd of people cheering us in. Carsten helped us both off the boat – Christ, the pier felt wobbly. I just had to stand still after stepping off the boat and clasp my quads as I tried to get used to being on land, and plucking up the courage to take my first steps. I was fully prepared to face-plant into the deck.

Steve made his way to Corina – I couldn't see Dad. Feeling very disorientated, I could make out Darryl and Sean from Two-Inna-Row, who were directly ahead, so I lurched towards them and hugged it out.

It was then that I heard someone calling out: Dad. That hug was magical, and I definitely needed that from someone I loved and greatly respected. Dad just told me over and over how proud he was, and the words made me feel like the king of the world. To say my legs were wobbly was an understatement – they somehow didn't feel attached to my body. I had to be incredibly careful as I then made my way over to Carsten to be interviewed along with Steve.

A few of the other competitors were there to greet us and administer hugs, too – Laura from Atlantic Girls, and Chris from Team Emotive. More words were exchanged with Two-Inna-Row. The rivalry was over; we started the journey as competitors and ended it as friends. Darryl was very croaky, having lost his voice on account of excess screaming and shouting to see us over the line.

We were then interviewed a couple of times – once by Carsten, and another by Charlotte. Carsten touched on the number of challenges we had during our row, and in an answer to one of his questions I started to list out all the things we'd faced, until Steve playfully reminded me that we were now trying to sell the boat.

Charlotte mentioned our general state of undress for most of the row, which was quite amusing. I was fully conscious that Rachel and the kids would be watching the live feed back home, so I made sure I let them know that I was thinking of them. They'd been a huge part of the team from the beginning, especially Rachel, and at that moment I really wish I could have shared it with them in person. Rachel in particular, who is terrified of ocean-based activities, had been part of the rowing club for a year, even completing the iconic Sark to Jersey row to show her support.

Due to the late nature of our arrival, it was close to 1am before we finally sat down for a burger and beer, courtesy of Atlantic Campaigns. Eating hot food and enjoying an ice-cold beer was certainly a welcome treat. Christ, they tasted good. Everyone was gradually dispersing, understandably, leaving us with Dad and Corina to catch up and tell them some stories about our journey. Given the fact that we were still wearing speedos, and my hair was particularly clown-like, we didn't think it was the right time to have a full-on party in the nearby nightclub. There was plenty of time for that later!

At about 1.30am, we departed to go our separate ways – Steve and Corina to their hotel, and me and Dad to our B&B. His unexpected but welcome appearance saved me from having to get Rachel to book somewhere for me – not to mention subsequently blagging a lift from somewhere!

The experience of being on level land, combined with my first beers in months, made me feel incredibly unsteady, to the point where I had to hold on to Dad's shoulders. Everything felt strange – even the car ride to the B&B felt odd, having a relatively non-bumpy journey. I gazed out of the window as Dad drove, just thinking how weird it was to be moving without manually powering the vessel. I'd also been worried about sea sickness before the race, with all the bumps associated with being at sea. Now, not being on it felt like an experience in itself.

The first thing I did when I got to the B&B was phone Rachel and the kids. I needed to do this on Dad's mobile, since the screen on my mobile was still shattered. I'd need to get that fixed in the coming days. I can't fully recall the conversation with Rach and the kids, but I was no doubt in full excitable babble mode. It was great to hear their voices, and I didn't really know where to start in relation to the row. I was still taking it in myself. Eventually, the call came to an end, and I had a happy wobbly-lipped moment as I reflected on how much I'd missed them.

From there, it was like one little victory after another. Having a shower! Getting water from a tap! Using an actual toilet, rather than a bucket! Things that previously I'd taken for granted now seemed like luxuries.

As I attempted with futility to drift off – in the absence of the rocking waves, the room seemed to be obligingly moving around instead – one thought kept floating through my mind.

I had done it.

I had rowed across the Atlantic Ocean.

For a couple of years, I'd found it hard to look beyond this moment. Now it had been reached.

What next?

Interlude 15.1

SEEING LAND was a wonderful experience. Despite anticipating it and being told that we'd see it around 20 miles out, it still somehow came as a surprise. I'd seen it over my shoulder first, and told Pete. He was busy rowing, so I carried on enjoying the far-off view. Pete wanted to finish his shift and enjoy it, as I had. With the anticipation building for him, I'm sure he was very disappointed when he was able to put the oars down and stand up, only to be greeted with absolutely nothing. The sun had now dipped behind the island, and clouds had gathered over Antigua, keeping it covered for a few more hours.

In the lead-up to this, we'd started seeing a lot more bird life, starting with the prehistoric, Pterodactyl-like frigatebirds seen in the vast distance, either fighting or flirting with each other. They were enormous, and could be seen from a mile or two away. We had a few small birds come and join us on the boat, which was nice. Marine life remained limited, but on the plus side, so did the anticipated rubbish. We witnessed very little flotsam and jetsam.

The final few hours were rather challenging, mainly as our ocean-rowing boat, designed for just that, was now needed as a coastal-rowing boat again, just as it had been in Jersey. Unfortunately, they're not designed for that, and she remained very difficult to control in the high tailwinds and short, sharp, steep waves. They were pushing us very favourably towards the island – and the rocks!

We hadn't had much of a briefing about the lay of the land around Antigua, so became a bit nervous as we approached this large, dark land mass in high winds and rough seas. All we could see were twinkling lights of various villages and dwellings, some more concentrated than others.

The charts showed lots of inlets and headlands and, from the angle we were approaching, we couldn't make out which inlet we needed to be heading for. There was also the question of admin: we needed to prepare our passports, documentation and SD/memory cards, and ensure that the Sat phone was on and ready to receive calls, along with the VHF. All navigation and searchlights had to be on, and we needed to dig out our flares, plus a bucket of water to extinguish them – all while rowing in very windy conditions in an unfamiliar area.

We managed, though, and as we rounded the headland of what seemed like the fifth inlet, we saw the small boats of the welcoming committee. I'd expected to get around the headland into the cove and be protected by the wind, but the opposite seemed to happen – it intensified with a plan to push us west and prevent us from finishing. With all my strength (and probably dreadful technique), we managed to get over the finish line for a big hug, a very British handshake, and some nice flare photography.

Steve Hayes

Interlude 15.2

ANTIGUA WAS a great final destination. I kind of wish we'd arrived during the day to fully appreciate the surroundings, colours, superyachts, honking horns from nearby boats and the azure waters, but it wasn't to be. Besides, the night-time finish photos with flares in hands are always pretty cool.

I'd watched every team for the past couple of years finish, so knew what to expect in terms of the race team coming out to greet us, the small crowds gathering, and shaking hands with Carsten and the rest of the crew. I knew to expect to be wobbly coming off the boat, but I still nearly fell over. I hugged a couple of other rowers that had come to greet us before seeing my wife for a tearful hug – hers, not mine!

As it was now the early hours of the morning, the crowds dispersed fairly quickly, leaving Pete and me awkwardly sitting in a very gusty gazebo in our budgie smugglers, chowing down on a burger and a beer. We went our separate ways to reconvene the next morning to clean and organise the boat. I'd spent a couple of hours catching up with my wife and sister-in-law at the accommodation, drinking and gawping at the size of my toddler, Sophia, stretched out and fast asleep diagonally across our bed.

Interestingly, a question we get asked a lot is what we missed the most. One thing that springs to mind is the temperature. During the row, after a week or so, when you make it far enough south, everything becomes the same temperature: the weather is warm, the water is warm, everything below the waterline of the boat matches the sea's temperature. Food and drinks are all the same temperature, whether it's beef jerky or a Snickers – it's all the same. Havana rum or desalinated sea water – nothing changes.

When I arrived at my accommodation for the night – a B&B up on a hill overlooking the bay we'd rowed into – I was guided towards an honesty bar with fridge and freezer. I opened the freezer door and was engulfed in a cold cloud of frigid air. I sat there for a few moments, enjoying a feeling I hadn't even realised I missed – the cold. It was a delight to add a few ice cubes to my large glass of rum.

The remaining days were spent being a tourist in Antigua and catching up with family and decompressing – and trying to get my phone repaired!

Steve Hayes

Chapter 16

Slaying dragons and playing with cars

THE YEARS 2018 and 2019 stand out for several reasons. On the one hand, there was the sheer number of challenges I'd decided to do for charity (more on the reasons for these later). On the other, our family received some pretty devastating news.

Towards the end of 2017, my mum had been back and forth with various consultants, who thought her symptoms might be just a case of her still recovering from a previous operation. As it turned out, this wasn't the case; just before the end of 2017, she was diagnosed with cancer of the gallbladder.

To make ever such a slight understatement, it's not a good one to have. Survival rates are 60 per cent – if it's found early. The trouble is, this doesn't usually happen; only 20 per cent of cases are spotted in the early stages. Obviously, if left untreated, the cancer is much more likely to spread. When this happens, the survival rate falls to just 2 per cent over the subsequent five years.

The early news didn't look good: the first consultant my mum and dad visited gave them the news quite heavy-handedly, seeming distinctly lacking in any kind of bedside manner, making it seem like her days were numbered (this particular medical professional was subsequently nicknamed 'Doctor Death').

There was no road map at all, and my parents were ushered out of the door after receiving the news. I recall their subsequent visit to Jersey just after Christmas, which was when they told us about the diagnosis. My dad was in pieces when we had a private chat about it shortly after. Seeing him like this was one of the hardest things I'd ever experienced.

Thankfully, later visits with other doctors showed that the cancer was treatable. Even so, with what was happening, I felt it best to inform my employers that I might be having to make some trips to the mainland in the near future. Having had my world rocked once already, I was unaware that this simple conversation would have profound ramifications.

On the career front, it's probably best that I rewind a bit. As I mentioned a while back, I'd been working for a precious metals business for eight years, and things had been going well. I'd joined in the very early days of the company, taken on a great deal of responsibility and thrived professionally as the business grew. Then, a takeover happened. Long story short, there was a new owner with very different ideas on how to run things, and my time at the company came to an end.

With a young family to support, I needed a job quickly, and ultimately ended up settling for one in a bank. While it filled a gap, I knew from day one in the office that it really wasn't what I wanted to do, and I was looking for an exit route more or less from the beginning. However, I didn't fancy being unemployed again, so I simply got my head down while seeking other opportunities.

I duly found this in the form of a vacancy at a small company in the Jersey finance industry. It was a bit of a risk – a six-month contract, with no guarantee of being kept on at the end. While I couldn't see myself in this role long-term, it at least had the benefit of being secure and, again, I had a family to support. Despite this, I took the plunge, and in the summer of 2016 stepped into a new role, knowing full well that half a year later I might be back to square one, with my CV looking a bit suspect.

Ultimately, it all worked out pretty well – I enjoyed the work, which was challenging and varied, and with it being a small company there was always plenty to get stuck into. A couple of months after starting, the boss called me into the office and asked what I thought about making it a full-time arrangement. Happy days – I immediately agreed.

Work carried on in this vein, and I got on well with the boss, who it felt like was constantly singing my praises as I successfully turned my hand to various projects within the business. Even then, however, with things seemingly going well, I couldn't shake off a sense of unease, as I'd witnessed things going south for some people who had been flavour of the month previously, even to the extent that they felt they had no other options but to leave the business.

When he turned on someone – which seemed to happen quickly, and often at random – there seemed to be little to be done. But I didn't give it a huge amount of thought beyond that – I was doing fine, after all, but his treatment of others didn't sit well with me at all.

However, over time, my negative feelings grew. I had this spider sense about feeling nervous about my role, like his attitude towards me was changing a bit. I wasn't quite sure what was going on. Would I be next?

Then, I got the news about Mum. Immediately after that, I went to see my boss to let him know the situation, and that I might have to make some trips to the UK in the coming year, depending on how things went. He was very nice about it all – very supportive, as you'd expect people to be – and left me feeling as okay as I could be about everything.

The next day, he called me into his office. Before I knew what was going on, he absolutely tore into me. The reason for his anger was something that was: a) incredibly minor, and b) something I hadn't even done.

I was baffled – even if it was something that I *had* done, he'd have had an idea of where I was emotionally after our conversation the previous day. What sort of person does that?

As later events showed, this wasn't a one-off. From that point on, it became a case of pulling me up for every single thing I did. While before, I'd been the golden child, incapable of getting anything wrong, now I was permanently on the receiving end, with duties being taken away from me. I found it embarrassing and humiliating, and it was a case of, *Okay, I might not have a future in this business. This is just what I need.*

I was taking a bit of outside legal advice from a friend, making note of dates, times, conversations, etc., so I could prepare my case if it came to it, but I needed something else to focus on. As luck would have it, I had 'the Ice Ultra (see Chapter 14), which gave me the perfect opportunity to get out of there, focus a bit and clear my head.

I remember being out there in the day stages, clear snow and sky all around me, almost like a blank canvas. *When I get home, I need to take control of this situation.* Everything felt simple – it was the moment of clarity that I needed. The other thought I had as I looked across the snow was imagining a giant polar bear savaging my then-boss, while making it clear he had no designs on me.

When I got back home to Jersey, I got straight to it: I went in and asked him directly what his problem was. I phrased it thus: 'I have the distinct impression that you might have an issue with me. Do you mind explaining what it is?'

Explain he did – reeling off lots of unfounded accusations from his imaginary parchment in the process. The paradox here was that his PA happened to also have responsibility for HR at the company. While my immediate thought was that it could be a conflict of interest in getting any kind of meaningful justice, his PA tried to find a way we could work together, and was very fair.

In the end, the conclusion was that the two of us should have more frequent dialogue and iron out our differences that way. By this stage, I didn't have any confidence that this approach would be successful, so I responded, 'Well, that could be an option, or we could come to another form of agreement,' and that's what happened.

The last few days were odd, as an announcement was put out about me leaving, but I had to hang around for a few days, obviously unable to disclose anything. Colleagues would understandably come up to me and ask me where I was going. My stock response was, 'I have no new role,' which always brought wide-eyed responses. I sometimes played around with the response and said, 'To pursue a career as a male model,' or, 'Become an astronaut,' to make light of the situation. Nevertheless, I walked out of there – unemployed again, and took myself to the pub on my one-man leaving do!

Interestingly, this new era led on to something quite novel for me: my first studio TV appearance. The local newspaper had run an article on me competing in the Ice Ultra. The day it came out, I got a call from ITV – they'd read the article, and had a gap in their schedule that needed doing, and asked if I wanted to go on that evening. Sure, why not?

Rachel was at work, and I happened to have the kids with me, so I took them both to the studio. Having not thought about it previously, as I sat and waited for my turn, I started to feel a tad nervous. *I'm going to be on TV.*

A conversation with a runner later, and it turned out I'd misread the situation. Based on the phone conversation, I'd assumed that my talk would be pre-recorded. Nope, it transpired that I'd be speaking live on TV. Gulp.

Leila chose that time to helpfully interject: 'Are you nervous Daddy? Is your face going to go pink?' Just what I needed – the ringing endorsement of my daughter before I went live on air! Thankfully, it all went well.

In light of Mum's news, and me finding myself with more time on my hands, my way of dealing with these new circumstances was consistent with how I'd approached the previous few years in Jersey: doing a lot of silly endurance challenges!

This is how I first got involved with Macmillan, who I've now actively fundraised for over several years. While they themselves weren't involved with Mum's care, I wanted to support a charity that was both local and involved with helping people with cancer. To this end, I introduced myself to them, explained my background – using the Ice Ultra as a recent example – and underlined my plan: to participate in and devise numerous challenges – possibly one a month – and simply raise as much as I can.

Having left the job, after a very short period of elation it dawned on me what a car crash my career had been for the last two or three years. I had a bit of a crisis of confidence and was hitting some lows, so decided to regain control. I started this with my first event of the new regime: the Transylvania 100.

This was one that had been suggested to me by Steve, who had done it previously (coincidentally, it's also where his wife, Corina, is from).

While Steve had a decent track record in suggesting challenges, I was having a bit of a wobble – my confidence still hadn't recovered, and I wasn't training well at all. Plus, I didn't fancy the idea of wandering off and getting lost in the Romanian mountains. (Steve probably shouldn't have mentioned to me that when he did it the previous year, at one point he got lost and ended up getting attacked by gypsies and wolves

– not sure if they were separate incidents, or at the same time.)

I laid bare my concerns, and Steve's response was simple: we'd do it together. He dragged me out there, we did the event and it was brilliant fun – just what I needed, to get out and get challenged a bit. We did most of the event together until about ten miles from the end. Steve was moving much better than me, so I told him to jog on and that I'd finish it on my own. It was perfect: spectacular, mountainous scenery and a bit of snow, all set to a backdrop of seemingly unending wilderness. As an added bonus, we didn't get attacked by anything this time. This event really brought me back to life a bit, and something positive was happening on the job-hunting front.

The job hunt hadn't been going as planned, and while in the build-up to the event I'd been focusing my thoughts on that, I was able to get a lot of my confidence back. Fairly soon after I got home, I was offered a new job, and accepted it. At the time of writing, I'm still there.

From then on, up until the end of 2018, I took on numerous other challenges, among them the Round Island Challenge (a 48-mile run), Round the Rock (another 48-mile run), Coast to Coast (a 145-mile non-stop run from Whitehaven to Tynemouth) the Breca Swimrun (a 33-mile non-stop sea swim/run combination), the Jersey Marathon (ran while hungover after a day on the beers with my visiting brothers – not a recommended approach), and the Dorset Marathon (a spectacular jaunt along the Purbecks – and one that first planted the seed in my mind of getting a springer spaniel as a running partner).

The final challenge of the year was an idea formed by Steve, which he called 'Through the Gears'. The aim was to start cycling at noon on New Year's Eve around a one-mile circuit and keep going into New Year's Day, non-stop for 24 hours. I decided to join Steve on the challenge with a week's notice. At this point, I didn't even own a suitable bike, so Richard Tanguy at Big Maggy's Bike Shop in Jersey lent me one. I was also away in the UK at Christmas, arriving back on 30 December, so had one day to get familiar with the bike, to include clipping in, which is something I'd never done before. It was an interesting and rather painful experience, but I managed in the region of 350 miles. Steve was excellent, managing well over 400 miles.

It all felt very rewarding, getting back to what I enjoyed: challenging myself and continuing to push onwards. It also helped me deal with what was happening to Mum: she was going through increasingly gruelling stages of treatment and was an absolute inspiration to me. She always maintained her sense of humour, and it pushed me to want to continue to fundraise for a local charity that helped others like her.

So with my 2018 list of challenges complete, I met with Macmillan and told them I was coming up with a list for 2019. Since these were follow-on challenges, it seemed only natural that I should be trying to raise the bar, and this would certainly be the case with the final challenge of 2019, and more on this shortly.

The challenges in 2019 started with the Macmillan rowathon, which is a 30km row on a Concept2 rowing machine as a team of five. There's a morning and afternoon session to cater for all teams entered. I decided to do both sessions consecutively and solo – so 60km non-stop on a Concept2. Little did I know that, a few years later, I'd be rowing a slightly longer distance.

The challenges this year continued and included Dragon's Back, the Wendover Woods 100-mile ultra run, and a 24-hour non-stop indoor cycle ride, which took place at Jersey's Super League Triathlon. The Dragon's Back was particularly satisfying, as I was able to fully exorcise the demons of 2015, where I'd quit at the end of day one. This time around, head in the game and knowing full well what to expect (and having trained accordingly), I managed to slay the dragon.

My final event of 2019 – and one of the more unique challenges I ended up completing – came about as a result of a visit home. Back in Dorset, while paying a visit to Mum and Dad at some point in 2018, the local news was on, with something about a guy called Ross Edgley, who had run a marathon while pulling a mini.

Most people's reaction: what a nutter.

My reaction: what a great idea.

From that moment on, I couldn't think of anything else. I'd been looking for major fundraising ideas that would generate a significant amount, and this was perfect. It would test me in ways I hadn't been tested before, and I was pretty sure that no one in Jersey had done it.

The car to be towed was a Smart car provided by the wonderful man that is Derrick Slatter, who would go on to become our title sponsor for the Atlantic row. There may be mischievous smiles about it being just a Smart car, but it still weighed just under a ton, and for a large part of the challenge I'd also have a person sitting in the car steering, adding to this weight.

Having worked out a route, which consisted of out and backs along a section of Jersey's five-mile road, and agreed it with the relevant parishes, of which there were three, I duly managed it!

Tough and incredibly painful was an understatement, and I instantly regretted my decision not to over-inflate the tyres on the day of the challenge as I pulled this hunk of metal, via a harness, over a very unforgiving road surface. The day's agony paled by the fact I was so well supported by Rachel, friends and the wider community: £20,000 was raised.

It marked a big change for me – focusing on strength training rather than the usual cardio – but it all turned out okay, and the most important muscle, as always, was the mind and the will to complete it. The success of this challenge was in many ways thanks to Dan Garrido, a friend and personal trainer who took me under his wing free of charge and coached me for quite a few months. I learned an awful lot from Dan, and have taken this into many subsequent challenges.

While I don't do these challenges for any kind of recognition, it has drawn attention in places, as well as the surprising but flattering focus from another area.

The Pride of Jersey Awards aims to showcase the amazing community spirit that's such an important feature of island life. I've been privileged enough to be nominated twice – first for Best Fundraiser in 2020, and again in 2023 for Ambassador of the Year (which I won!). Steve also got in on the action, as we took home the winning prize in the 'Local Hero' category at the awards.

Among all of these, there were the challenges that got away. One example was swimming the English Channel – I'd seen it done, and never contemplated being able to achieve it. Naturally, it had to be attempted. While I'm not one to shy away from a challenge, there were certain aspects of it that didn't appeal to me. First off, it's recommended that you gain quite a bit of weight in preparation. It was necessary, but I didn't relish the physical transformation that was required. Even so, I carried on practising.

However, fates conspired against me. On 23 March 2020, the first national lockdown in the UK for the COVID-19 pandemic was announced. With all the swimming pools on the island shut, I was limited in where I could practise – the sea was my only option. While this was fine at certain times of year, at others it became far too cold to stay out there for the amount of time I needed to, bearing in mind I was training in just my speedos with no wetsuit. Those times hobbling shivering back to the car, futilely trying to unlock the car as my frozen, claw-like hands fumbled with the keys, will live long in the memory.

I got as far as completing the six-hour qualifying swim required to compete (putting up with an unwelcome jellyfish sting to the face), but I never took up the place. As I increased my training distance significantly and attempted a ten-hour swim, I injured my rotator cuff and had to defer my place, and ultimately never did take it up.

Plus, I had a proposal from Steve on another water-based challenge to focus my attention on.

Interlude 16.1

SURPRISE, PRIDE and sometimes downright fear are probably the most applicable words that describe how Carol and I have felt about Pete's relatively later-life journey from occasional jogger to ocean rower.

As a kid, Pete was always outgoing and determined. Like most lads, he liked football and outdoor pursuits, but was frequently hampered by some distant genes that left him prone to hay fever and asthma, and he needed to carry an inhaler at all times to help with the latter.

Two particular episodes from his childhood illustrate the challenges he faced. Having looked forward to his first camping trip with the Cubs for months, he had to abandon it before the first day was out because he was in such a bad way with his hay fever. Similarly, a family holiday to Cornwall during a particularly rainy summer saw Pete developing bronchitis, and us having to cut the trip short and hurriedly get him home for some medical care.

As Pete reached his teens and early manhood, a lot of his earlier childhood health problems cleared up, although the asthma and need for the inhaler unfortunately didn't go entirely. As I remember these years, Pete started occasional visits to the gym with his mates, and started jogging as well. I don't remember any of this being too serious in those days, although I did note that he appeared to enjoy jogging, which I, and more certainly his mother, never did.

When Pete told us he intended to enter his first marathon run, we weren't too surprised, because he was already following the classic route of runs over progressively longer distances, and clearly enjoyed competing. After a successful finish and a few more marathons, the ultramarathons started to come along as well.

To be honest, we didn't see this development coming. We never doubted that Pete had the determination and mental strength that are essential to compete in these kinds of endurance events, but as he has since shown, he'd also developed the necessary physical strength and resilience as well. It was some consolation to us that these subsequent races appeared to be well organised. However, day and night, and sometimes non-stop races over crazy distances through deserts, jungles, Arctic snows, and snow-clad mountain ranges inevitably carried all manner of dangers with them, so the best bits for us were always when it had been confirmed that Pete had finished safely.

I remember taking the phone call from Pete when he broke it to me that his next jaunt would be to row the Atlantic with his mate, Steve. He was clearly bubbling, but all I could think of was how to break this news to his mum, and that this would involve far more risks than anything he'd done before. As worried as I was, however, and remained throughout, I knew we had to do all we could to support him, as clearly the decision was already made. Nearly three years later, as the clock approached midnight local time, I found myself waiting on the dockside in English Harbour, Antigua, along with other assorted family members, mates, fellow racers and officials. Finally, the flares lit up, and we saw DragonFish appear out of the distant gloom, with Pete and Steve sensibly clutching bottles of just-opened champagne.

My abiding memories from this evening were just how relieved and thankful I felt that they'd both made it home safe and well. This was tempered just a bit by my concerns about just how skinny they both looked, with Pete in particular having lost well over three stone. Finally, there were my first words to Pete when we embraced for the first time on the quayside after the official landing ceremony: 'If you ever think of doing anything like this again then I will ******* strangle you.'

Jack and Carol Wright, Pete's parents

Interlude 16.2

MY HUSBAND is not your average adventure enthusiast. Over the years, he has tackled some of the most extreme endurance challenges imaginable, including rowing the Atlantic, running a marathon while pulling a car, and participating in events like the Marathon des Sables, Jungle Marathon, Ice Ultra and Ultra Trail du Mont Blanc, and these don't even scratch the surface.

Each time he commits to one of these, I find myself both amazed and exhausted, knowing that while he's out there pushing his limits, I'm the one holding down the fort back home. It's not easy juggling all the household responsibilities, especially when he returns shattered and I'm ready to pass his half of the chores back. In the beginning, I was much more patient, but now I tell him straight: 'This is your idea of fun, you still have to do your bit at home!' I'm not sure what he finds harder: the excruciating pain and exhaustion from completing these crazy challenges, or returning home to a moany and stressed-out me!

We met during a job interview back in 2001, and instantly clicked, becoming friends. We mucked about at work so much that I was forced to move desks when he went on holiday! After a couple of years of trying (and failing) to set him up with friends, we started dating and never looked back. We've been married for 18 years now, and in that time we've raised two fantastic children. We've always valued family stability while supporting each other's hobbies and adventures.

He wasn't a runner when we met – just a very good partying companion, but when the kids came along he ditched weekend hangovers for weekend runs. He signed up for the London Marathon, and never looked back. It took him a few tough years of injuries to get there, which was difficult to watch, but in true Pete fashion he doubled down, pulled up his big-boy pants and made sure he got to the start line. Every new race he did, he'd meet someone who had done something different that would spark his interest, and he'd be signed up to something new before he landed back in Jersey.

Living with an ultrarunner, it's hard not to catch the running bug. I'm no runner, but had decided that I wanted to run just one marathon before I turned 40. Pete promised to run it with me, and we found the Polar Circle Marathon in Greenland, which ticked every box for me, and even had an extra half-marathon that he could do so he could scratch his ultra run itch at the same time. We started on a stunning glacier, and he encouraged me every step of the way, even managing to stay calm while I had a diva dip halfway through that may have had a few tears and snot involved! It's one of my favourite memories, and I'll cherish it forever. I couldn't be more proud of Pete. His commitment, resilience and the sheer drive he has for his adventures are awe-inspiring.

Another favourite of mine was when Pete and Steve took on the Jungle Marathon and were raising funds for Durrell Wildlife Trust. Henry Cavill is an ambassador for the charity, as he is from Jersey, and the boys had a photoshoot with him to help boost their profile. There was absolutely no way I was going to miss that, so I gate-crashed the meeting, with two young children in tow as an excuse. We got a photo taken, and I definitely held on a bit too long when holding on to him, but there has to be some perks to being an ultrarunner's wife!

However, there have been moments when his challenges tested my patience. One of the most difficult times was during the COVID-19 pandemic when Pete decided to run increasing hours each day to match the date of the month, all while raising money for Macmillan, a cause close to his heart due to his mother's illness. While I admired his dedication, the combination of home-schooling, working full-time and dealing with a zombie-like runner took its toll. After he completed the challenge, I snapped, reminding him in screaming banshee style that he still had responsibilities at home! Once I got it off my chest, the tension lifted, but Pete was hurt and upset for a few days, because he'd been so proud of his achievement. The hurt soon became a transformation to super-nice and thoughtful, so I should have known something was going on!

Unbeknownst to me, Pete's equally 'challenging' friend, Steve, had been in touch, looking for a partner to row the Atlantic with! A very sheepish Pete did the bravest thing I've ever seen him do, and raised the idea with me of him doing the race in two years' time. Despite thinking it was a ridiculous idea, I agreed to support him, and he signed up before I could change my mind. I even took up rowing myself, thinking we might spend some time together rowing, forgetting for a short time how focused my husband gets when he has an idea in his head. I joined a novice group instead at the Jersey Rowing Club, and we completed the Sark to Jersey race. Did I mention that my team beat Pete and Steve?

By November 2022, Pete and Steve were setting off for La Gomera to row the Atlantic. The kids and I waved them off, but on the way back, I stopped in London for an angiogram. I'd found out earlier in the year that I had a couple of brain aneurysms, and while Pete was away I learned that surgery would be necessary. We scheduled it for February, just a week after Pete returned from his triumphant journey. I had a bit of time to get him to the barbers and try to fatten him up before I left. The kids and I particularly enjoyed knocking on the wall when he was sleeping, upon which he'd jump up and start rowing in bed. That one definitely never got old! His arrival home coincided with his 50th birthday but, instead of celebrating, I was preparing for surgery. I still feel guilty that I couldn't give him the celebration he deserved, although my sister insists that surviving the surgery was a pretty special birthday gift!

Through it all, Pete has continued to amaze me with his perseverance and courage, and while his adventures may test my patience at times, I couldn't be prouder of everything he's achieved.

Rachel Wright, Pete's wife

Epilogue

FOR ALL the euphoria of finally completing an endeavour that was several years in the making, there's always something waiting to bring you crashing back down to earth. This arrived the next morning, when I had to do the absolute last thing I felt like: go back to the boat!

Thankfully, it wasn't a return journey; we had to get it clean and ready for shipment back to the UK. It was just as well that we were getting this out of the way – it was absolutely filthy. As much as we'd tried to keep on top of things on the cleanliness front, there was plenty of accumulated grime from our nearly two months at sea. Probably some remnants of flying fish, too.

Still feeling very wobbly on land, the moment I set foot back on the boat, everything felt right again. It was incredibly surreal. Maybe the sailor's life was for me after all?

Scratch that thought.

The clean-up operation took most of the morning. Once that was done, I spent some time catching up with Dad. He'd helped us out early on in the race with a loan to fund the deposit on the boat, which was invaluable, since we hadn't secured any sponsors at that point. At the same time, he'd also voiced his concern about the challenge and sworn me to secrecy in relation to disclosing his involvement to Mum. (Mum, now you know, it all turned out okay!) Dad had had to wait around in Antigua for quite a few days due to our delayed arrival, so it meant a lot to have him here.

The following day, Dad 'surprised' me by taking me on a scenic hike he'd discovered. I wasn't so enthusiastic about this, even when he mentioned that there was a great viewing point of the harbour. However, his casual mention of a nearby bar sold it to me.

It was only during this relatively short hike that I realised how much of a physical toll the race had taken on me – even this two-mile stroll was an effort. Calf muscles – gone. Arm muscles – gone. Hamstrings – incredibly weak. On the plus side, my back, shoulders and quads were all incredibly strong, so there was that. Looks like I had some muscle to build back in the coming months.

Upon reaching the bar after a gruelling 45-minute ascent, we discovered that it was closed. It wasn't quite a Charlton Heston in *Planet of the Apes* 'damn it all to hell!' moment, but it was a near thing.

Shorn of any access to social media due to the destruction of my phone, it was impossible to gauge the level of support from everyone back home. I had to rely on Dad's mobile to chat to Rachel and the kids while my phone was sent off to have the screen repaired courtesy of our lovely landlady. It was only when I headed back to Atlantic Campaigns HQ after the hike for an interview from various media in Jersey that I started to appreciate the level of support we'd had. It was incredibly humbling, knowing all the people that had been tracking us, supporting us and donating to our nominated charities. I hadn't quite expected this after we made unflattering headlines in the local newspaper during our final training row! It just served to make everything all the more fulfilling and worthwhile.

While I enjoyed the slower pace, feeling the land beneath my feet, getting a decent amount of sleep, and the post-race atmosphere, it didn't feel right without Rachel and the kids. I'd been away a long time and sacrificed a lot of time with them, not only during the race itself, but in the build-up. Making up for this was at the top of my priority list.

Plus, Rachel had a date for her operation booked in. I also wanted to get back in time to celebrate our wedding anniversary on 8 February. In the event, the operation was a success, and at the time of writing she's progressing nicely.

So what was next? Recovery, obviously! The row had taken its toll, and while I'm not normally one for sitting still, even I recognised the need for some time out.

It was back to the day job, too. My employers had been incredibly understanding in letting me do this, and I'll always be grateful to them for that. Nevertheless, I needed to get back and start earning again, so I was back at work within a few days.

My employers' consideration extended to a surprise gift when I got back – on my first trip to the gents, I noticed a bucket hanging up on the door, bearing the message 'Peter Wright: Sole Use'. Very kind of them to ease my transition away from sea life!

In the weeks and months that followed my return to Jersey and day-to-day life, I've reflected on a few things.

In terms of how it measured up to the race I had in my head, if anything, it was far tougher and scarier than I ever imagined – and I'd imagined both in equal measure. I hadn't expected the level of equipment malfunction that we experienced, and certainly hadn't anticipated being stuck in the stern cabin for nearly five days. I was out of my comfort zone most of the time, but I always gave 100 per cent, was focused and revelled in the fact that I was actively living out something I'd dreamed about, and sharing the experience at the same time with a good mate.

Physically, I was in good shape beforehand, and in this respect, apart from a permanent sore bum, held it together pretty well. However, mentally it was in many ways tougher than I imagined, because the ocean has its own designs on you, and there's so much that's out of your control.

What did I get out of it? In life, we can all be our own worst critic, and I'm as guilty as the next person of that. On the ocean, I learned the power of self-praise in relation to problem-solving and working together, and the whole experience has made me more confident in relation to trying out new things. I also reflected on the version of me prior to 2013 (when I did the MDS) that would never have even entertained such a challenge, or in fact many others that I've done post-2013. I realised how much I've loved having a challenge that pushed the boundaries, and the positive effect it has had on my wellbeing and outlook in life. I was also able to continue to fundraise for local charities, and the £50,000 raised as a result of the row took total fundraising past the £100,000 mark since 2012.

What was the impact on my friendship with Steve? We were good mates before the row, and one of our joint goals was to keep it that way. Our goals had been to complete the challenge, stay mates, achieve our fundraising targets and not financially bankrupt ourselves. In 54 days, we had two very small arguments, and even during those we were just being honest with each other – sometimes that's what true friendship is all about. We didn't know what versions of our usual selves we'd become out on the ocean, and had to resolve to find ways of getting the best out of each other for as long as it took. We had so many laughs out there, and often chose to sacrifice sleep and just hang out on deck together. It's safe to say that my friendship with Steve is firmly intact.

The challenge was definitely life-affirming. From inception, Steve and I needed to learn many skills, notably learning to row, creating a company and brand, marketing it to secure £125,000 in sponsorship, ongoing project management, as well as the numerous other skills needed to make it to the start line. The major defining thing for me is the sheer magnitude of the challenge and the fact you row away from a tiny island with a vast expanse of unpredictability before you reach Antigua. It's mind-boggling, and I still pinch myself about being one of those who has successfully crossed an ocean. I guess I feel less daunted about other challenges moving forwards now!

What did I enjoy most out of it? Living in La Gomera for two weeks prior to the row was amazing, although blotted by homesickness. It was such a great atmosphere, and I guess a very different version of living in an Olympic village prior to the big event. I think I'll always feel a positive and emotional attachment to La Gomera, as well as Atlantic Campaigns and all the rowers I've had the pleasure of meeting.

In terms of the actual row, it was a cross between the tranquillity of a sunrise versus rowing under the stars. The stars win by a margin, and on many of my night shifts, as I felt at one with the ocean, I could find myself getting lost in the stars. The shooting star I witnessed falling through the sky will particularly live long in the memory.

As for what's next? Post-row, I decided to steer clear of challenges, but I felt like something very positive was missing. In 2024, I decided to take on the Centurion Grand Slam Challenge, which consisted of four 100-mile ultramarathons within five months of each other, and successfully completed this challenge.

My next big challenge, due October 2025, is to take on seven Iron Man distance triathlons in seven consecutive days on my home island of Jersey, and in turn raise more funds for local charities.

Will I row again? Maybe. I'll get back to you on that one! There are four more oceans, after all …

Acknowledgements

Pete:

This book began through a collection of blogs I'd scribbled down, and as the rowing adventure gained traction, I knew there was a story that I wanted to tell. I reflected more in numerous, sweaty, sleep-deprived moments in the stern cabin of our ocean-rowing boat over 54 days, and thought a lot about the timeline and events that had led to the situation I was in.

My addiction to endurance events effectively began with Marathon des Sables in 2013, and I have to give thanks to my friend Paul Burrows for his relentlessness in persuading me to take the plunge. I've never looked back, and completing the event was like opening Pandora's box. Throughout this event and all those that have followed, I've had the pleasure of meeting and being inspired by so many incredible people. Such individuals have included fellow runners, physios, coaches, nutritionists and personal trainers. Unfortunately, I can't name them all, but they most certainly know who they are.

Further thanks go to Tom Innes from the *Jersey Evening Post*, who has been a great supporter of ours. Both for keeping the public informed about our progress, and for giving us the privilege of a front page, we are grateful.

A special shout out, too, to Jim O'Garra, a local film producer in Jersey, who we approached at the beginning of the rowing project. Jim subsequently produced a 20-minute film about our row, which we titled, *An Oarsome Friendship*.

You can watch it here on Vimeo: bit.ly/ anoarsomefriendship

This book wouldn't have come to print without my baby brother, Steve. He spent a few days with me in La Gomera just before the row, which settled my nerves, and it was here that the 'book' idea was conceived. Steve then invested hours reading various books written by endurance athletes and pitching ideas on how to put it together. The result is what you've just read, and I'm immensely grateful to Steve for his support and in absolute awe of his editing skills.

My mum and dad have been a constant support throughout my life, and I've been lucky to spend so many special moments with them. My dad's work ethic, generosity and ability to turn his hand to seemingly anything particularly stand out as qualities I admire. As for my mum, her devilish sense of humour and her incredible fight and bravery in overcoming the odds in her battle with cancer served – and continue to serve – as an inspiration.

My sister Anna and brother Alan have always been checking in with me before races and challenges, and while my endeavours may have taken them by surprise and perhaps worried them both, they've always been an invaluable support, and made it clear that they're proud of me. Such sibling support has always made me feel stronger when facing challenges.

Of course, there is Steve Hayes. Pre-row, the challenges we tackled together simply wouldn't have been as fun or eventful without him. He's without doubt my endurance hero and principal influencer, having witnessed what he's done over the years, sometimes adopting rather suspect and unorthodox methods of training. It was an honour to have shared the rowing project with Steve, and it's something I'll always look back on with immense pride.

Finally, eternal thanks to my amazing wife, Rachel. I've lost count of the number of times you've seen my Montgomery Burns-like form return from an adventure, and helped put me back together despite being full-on yourself with work, kids and dogs. My favourite event memory of all time is when we completed the 2014 Polar Circle Marathon. I was so proud of your stubborn determination and humour as we laughed and grimaced our way around the course. As I've continued to set the bar higher for each challenge I take on, I know the reason for that is that you won't let me fail, and would definitely have my back if I did. Such support simply gives me the confidence to try things out and be the best version of myself that I can. I know you've always idolised Wonder Woman, and I've been amazed and in awe of your fighting spirit in overcoming recent brain surgery, while continuing with your volunteering roles outside of full-time work. I think these actions have surpassed any of Diana Prince's achievements.

Steve:

As I write these words, I can finally reflect on just how big a journey this book has been. From start to end, the process has taken roughly the same amount of time as Pete's preparation for rowing the Atlantic – thankfully, I didn't have to emulate his feat!

As it turned out, working on this book has been a life-changing time for me – during the time the book was being put together, I became both a husband and a father. To this end, my thanks go to my wife, Katherine, for her support as I partook in the plate-juggling exercise that was combining my first flailing experience of parenthood with shepherding this book towards publication, and patience in giving me the time I needed when time was in short supply. Furthermore, she was happy to cast a critical eye over the pages as they came in, spotting many a typo that had eluded me, and providing a great many suggestions that have ultimately made it a better book.

The biggest thanks of all go to the people who have provided the means for this book to exist: everyone at Pitch Publishing. I'll be forever grateful to you for affording me the opportunity to let this book see the light of day, and for humouring my (hopefully only occasionally frantic-sounding) emails.

A shout-out must also go to every race organiser who has answered my queries or let us use photos. Atlantic Campaigns in particular stand out in this regard, never letting something as trifling as organising the world's most difficult row get in the way of responding to my every enquiry promptly and with great candour.

Lastly – and very much not least – thanks, Pete. Echoing what I said at the start, it's been one hell of a journey (probably not as gruelling as your row, but hey ho!), and one that's been a privilege to be a part of.

Being able to show Theo what his Uncle Pete gets up to is something I can't wait to do, and seeing you and Rachel juggle parenthood while achieving everything you have gives me something to aim for myself. Thanks for everything.

Logic

for Information Technology

Logic

for Information Technology

Antony Galton
Exeter University, UK

JOHN WILEY & SONS

Chichester · New York · Brisbane · Toronto · Singapore

Other Wiley Editorial Offices

John Wiley & Sons, Inc., 605 Third Avenue,
New York, NY 10158–0012, USA

Jacaranda Wiley Ltd, G.P.O. Box 859, Brisbane,
Queensland 4001, Australia

John Wiley & Sons (Canada) Ltd, 22 Worcester Road,
Rexdale, Ontario M9W 1L1, Canada

John Wiley & Sons (SEA) Pte Ltd, 37 Jalan Pemimpin 05-04,
Block B, Union Industrial Building, Singapore 2057

Library of Congress Cataloging-in-Publication Data:

Galton, Antony.
    Logic for information technology / Antony Galton.
        p. cm.
    Includes bibliographical references and index.
    ISBN 0 471 92777 5 — ISBN 0 471 92933 6   (pbk)
        1. Logic, Symbolic and mathematical.   I. Title.
    QA9.G185   1990
    511.3—dc20   90-12446
                                                             CIP

British Library Cataloguing in Publication Data:
Galton, Antony *1952*
    Logic for information technology.
    1. Mathematics
    I. Title
    511.3

    ISBN 0 471 92777 5
    ISBN 0 471 92933 6 pbk

Typeset by Thomson Press (India) Ltd, New Delhi
Printed and bound in Great Britain by
Biddles Ltd, Guildford and King's Lynn